ANGEL HEALING

Claire Nahmad has published a number of books on healing, herbalism, magic and folklore. She lives in North Lincolnshire, England.

Love Spells
Cat Spells
Garden Spells
Dream Spells
Fairy Spells
Earth Magic
Magical Animals
The Enchanted Garden
The Cat Herbal
The Book of Peace
The Fairy Pack
Summoning Angels
The Secret Teachings of Mary Magdalene
    (With Margaret Bailey)
Your Guardian Angel

ANGEL HEALING

INVOKING THE HEALING POWER OF THE
ANGELS THROUGH SIMPLE RITUAL

CLAIRE NAHMAD

WATKINS PUBLISHING
LONDON

This edition first published in the UK in 2008 by
Watkins Publishing, Sixth Floor, Castle House,
75–76 Wells Street, London W1T 3QH

Reprinted 2009

3 5 7 9 10 8 6 4 2

Designed and typeset by Jerry Goldie

Printed and bound in Great Britain

British Library Cataloguing-in-Publication data available

ISBN: 978-1-905857-37-1

www.watkinspublishing.co.uk

CONTENTS

This book is dedicated
to Lisa Waugh, 'Brigid's Mirror'

ACKNOWLEDGEMEMTS

Acknowledgements are due to the White Eagle Lodge, London (tel. +44 [0]20 7603 7914) for their kind permission to quote material from publications by White Eagle; to Margaret Bailey, for permitting me to quote material from our book, *The Secret Teachings of Mary Magdalene*; and to Geoffrey Hodson, for his invaluable inspiration and guidance.

THE ANGELS OF
THE HEALING ART

The healing angels – under their mighty head, the Archangel Raphael – being filled with love for their human brethren, pursue their work continuously. Their presence by the sickbeds of men is a reality, though the minds and hearts of the majority of those responsible for healing of sickness are closed against them. Many who suffer and have suffered, know them well. They stand in their thousands on the spiritual and mental thresholds of every sickroom, in hospital or home, eager to enter in. Hitherto, but few have succeeded; the barriers upraised by human minds are often insuperable; should they break through these in spite of opposition, the precious healing which they bear in outstretched arms would be lost, dissipated in the effort to overcome resistance.

Hospitals and sickrooms could be filled with healing angels and healing power, if man would but spiritualize the healing art and regularly invoke spiritual and angelic healing help for the sick. If human minds can but be opened to these facts, the angel beside the bed of pain might become a far greater and far more living reality, whether in the private home or in great hospitals; and the whole work of healing and medical research might receive a tremendous impulse as the Archangel Raphael and his hosts descend amongst us and assist both in the healing of disease and in medical research.

Geoffrey Hodson

INTRODUCTION

The purpose of this book is to bring into focus the simplicity, serenity and beauty of angel healing. An excellent way to draw close to the angelic worlds and enjoy regular communion with the angels themselves, so that we begin to enjoy the innumerable benefits that such contact confers, is to actively engage with the angels in healing ourselves, one another and the planet. Angels are task-based, and the best way to invite them into our lives is to begin to work with them on a well-defined and practical basis.

As humanity attunes ever more deeply to the spiritual spheres, it will discover that the treatment of illness from the orthodox point of view, where the malaise is separated from its human context and bombarded with aggressive chemicals, becomes less and less satisfactory. A much wider scope of knowledge of our holistic being is required. The healing angels bear this knowledge, coming to us on exquisite colour rays which are aspects of consciousness itself. When we attune to the healing angels through simple and serene ceremony and ritual, healing floods our being on every level and releases us from the imprisonment of our sickness. We can then understand that the manifestation of our illness was a refusal, a blocked conduit, or a lack of understanding of the spiritual light which is our true essence.

My own experiences of communion with the angels led me to write my previous two books (*Summoning Angels* and *Your Guardian Angel*). I subsequently gave workshops on what I had personally experienced and learned in this field. The enthusiastic response and the number of spontaneous healings and angelic manifestations that took place during these workshops encouraged me to expand and intensify my focus on the path of angel therapy that was opening out before me, and I became eager to share with others the simple methods and procedures that the angels themselves were revealing to me. They are so easy to learn, so liberating and rewarding in their application and effects, it seemed to me that anyone could make use of them, even those among us who do not feel particularly attuned to the angelic realms!

There is nothing complicated about the healing rituals. Anyone, whether experienced in the subtleties of regular angelic contact or not, can put these simple healing ceremonies into operation at once, for their own benefit and the benefit of others. Although crystals, fragrances, flowers, coloured candles and other angelic correspondences are sometimes given in the text as an integral part of the healing ceremonies, the angels reassure us that our imagination is the key to successful ritual. You do not need to arm yourself with material paraphernalia before beginning to work with the angels.

I have made a point throughout of bringing to the fore certain methods of procedure which the angels themselves have requested, and which are essential in procuring and maintaining a strong, clear, highly functioning link with them. Many of these healing implementations spring from communications which I have received directly from angelic sources; others are the inspiration of that great angel seer, Geoffrey Hodson, one of the earliest of our present-day iconic angel teachers, to whom this book pays tribute. His teachings have always clarified and directed my understanding of my own communion with the angels.

The gentle techniques of angel healing outlined in the following pages will appeal to all those who seek deeper realities in the living of their lives than a purely materialistic philosophy can provide. Here is proof, growing ever clearer and more evident on a day-to-day basis as the healing rituals are put into practice, that angels do indeed exist and bear healing and transformation on their wings for the uplift and blessing of straitened humanity.

CHAPTER ONE

THE ANGEL OF THE POINTING HAND

In his book, *The Brotherhood of Angels and of Men*, Geoffrey Hodson gives us an evocative image of an angel pointing upwards – the 'angel of the pointing hand'. This image comprises the first lesson that the healing angels bring to us. We need to bear in mind always that the healing, inspiring, life-renewing domain of the angels cannot be entered at the level of ordinary, everyday awareness. We need to aspire heavenwards, to reach upwards in consciousness to the most exalted heights of which we can conceive. Simultaneously, we need to maintain a balance by realizing that our communion and cooperation with the healing angels takes place on the simplest level, in everyday circumstances, and, if we are to benefit fully, should indeed be a daily occurrence.

How can we reconcile these two apparently conflicting truths? Perhaps we can do so by embracing a new understanding of what we might term our 'everyday awareness'. Whilst we always need to be properly grounded in order to fulfil our earthly lives and to engage with mundane tasks, our corresponding mundane consciousness can be lifted many times throughout each day into a beautiful awareness of the angelic realms, so that communion with these beings becomes as natural as breathing, and our vision of life is no longer compressed into airless and stultifying compartments of dull materiality, but is shot through with the rainbow hues that are the dynamic joy and the soaring song of the angels.

Of course, it is all very well to wax lyrical about the angels in this vein, but how is that fine balance between operating in the mundane world and simultaneously inhabiting the beautiful angelic worlds achieved? It seldom happens of its own volition, especially as, through the increasing pressures and pace of 21st-century life and because of the nature of earthly incarnation, we are drawn into ever deeper and more concrete levels of materialism throughout the course of our lives. Moreover, our intellectual will cannot demand or summon it.

The angel of the pointing hand points upward with one hand, but the other hand stretches downward, grasping the head of the caduceus, that great symbol of opposite forces combining to create healing, harmony and wholeness upon the earth. Via this emblem, the angel closes his hand over ours, giving us the strength and inspiration to aspire to the highest, but keeping us firmly grounded and secure at the earthly level of our lives. These two aspects encompass the full meaning of the angel's message and teaching.

To enable us to achieve this state of balance, we can carry out the following exercises. They are a means of clearing the accumulated debris from the path of our spiritual will (that will within us which springs from the bidding of the heart, abiding always by its wisdom, and which uses aspiration, visualization and inner attunement to empower its objectives – never force).

Star Breathing

Sit quietly, and imagine a star of the purest white-silver taking radiant form in your heart. The star has six points.

Breathe in its brilliance, as if you drew each breath through your heart.

See yourself being slowly absorbed into its centre.

Rest easily in this exquisite star temple of the heart.

Feel the presence of the angels all around you.

The Spirit of the Rose

Relax, and imagine that you are sinking gently into the soft petals of a fragrant rose, the colour of the first flush of sunrise (ethereal pink with a muted and delicate red fire illuminating its depths).

Know that you are in the heart of the rose, and the rose is in your heart.

Feel its tender enfoldment, as if you were being drawn into the arms of a perfect love.

Inhale its beautiful perfume, which is the scent of paradise.

From it emerges the angel of the rose, like a dream given by the divine.

Breathe in the essence of this radiant angel, the quintessence of the rose, and let your spirit float, as if on air currents composed of the fragrance of the rose, into the shining higher realms.

The Ocean of Peace

Rest in the endless blue of a softly heaving ocean.

Breathe in its depths more easily, more invigoratingly, than you breathe air.

Feel the gentle, calming, cleansing rush of revitalization through your lungs as you take each breath of this magical element.

The water surrounds you with an eternal wash of

heavenly blue, but its waves are transparent and limpid as raindrops. They support you on a swelling breast of peace and wellbeing, the breast of motherhood and all that reassures.

Begin to realize that you are cradled within the heart of the great Angel of Peace. Her vibration is the sound of the white surf, infinitely hushed, and yet a huge sound, with a boom of might and majesty in it that soothes the ears and all the senses.

Sleep for a moment in the heart of this vast angel, and receive her healing in your bright dreams of ocean-deep peace.

Visionary Mountain

Think of the mountain tops, bathed in the golden glory of the sun.

Become aware of the soles of your feet treading the mountain heights with reverence, with worship. The Divine Presence dwells upon these shining hills.

Feel the freedom, the expanse of vision, the falling away of the fetters of little irritations and narrowness of perspective with which our earthly life can beset and burden us.

Let your vision take wing and soar as you walk upon the noble mountaintops.

Breathe the sparkling air that the angels breathe, and keep with you always this vast, clear, free-ranging vision from the mountains of the spirit.

Using these simple meditations, one or more for a few minutes each day, will help you to establish a strong and sure contact with the healing angels.

From time to time you may feel that your interior climate is dull and heavy, your heart closed, unresponsive and generally uninspired by the idea of angels! On these difficult days, it is probable that you stand in particular need of angelic healing, so it is well worth pursuing a few short and easy methods to dispel the inner clouds, and with them your rebelliousness and resistance to the programme of angel healing to which you have committed yourself. Our lower mind invariably attempts to scupper our best spiritual efforts, so its obtrusion necessarily means that you are making good progress and have achieved genuine and potent angelic contact, otherwise it wouldn't trouble itself to try to intervene! Here are three powerful exercises to get back on track. (Please note that when named angels are given in any exercise, it is always a good idea to call their name three times. This provides for a more powerful invocation.)

Petition to Vwyamus

Place yourself in the star of spiritual light. Ask the great cleansing angel Vwyamus (Vwy-ah-mus) to clear your surroundings and your aura of negative vibrations and accumulated psychic material. Vwyamus has power over the unpleasant etheric mucus that gathers in our immediate environment and within our auric field. This etherically viscous substance has the same effect as physical mucus in that it blocks our spiritual breathing and hearing passages, poisons our system and generally makes us feel off-colour! The dynamic cleansing and clearing virtues of Vwyamus dissolve and purify all forms of etheric mucus, absorbing it into the heart of high-spinning angelic energy so that its pollutants are transformed into golden etheric atoms charged with effervescent life-force. You can use the following invocation, or you may prefer to petition Vwyamus using your own words.

Great Angel Vwyamus

Cleanse me of all accumulated etheric mucus,

of all negative psychic matter that clings within

and to my aura and that pollutes my surroundings.

Cleanse me in the west, cleanse me in the east

cleanse me in the south, cleanse me in the north.

Encircle me with your power of cleansing,

your silver spinning loops that purge and clear.

Shed your purifying light throughout me

and all around me until I am immaculate.

Thank you, dear angel of the heights.

Be with me and shine in me throughout this day.

As with all angel work, we cannot expect everything to be done for us. Of course, the angels constantly perform marvels and wonders on our behalf; but they will never take on a role which might encourage us to cease our progression on our spiritual path and fall into a stupor by the wayside. They will always guard against our tendency to fall into atrophy, inertia and dependence.

When we work to clear negative conditions from our chakras, our aura and our environment, the angels will do it for us, especially if one or more of the methods outlined are utilized. A way will clear through the mists as they act upon our bidding, but we must be alert to it, and set our feet firmly on the shining trail that the angels reveal to us, prepared to use our own strength and determination to prevent the shadows from gathering again. Of course, if they do, we simply ask once more for the angels' help; but it is important to recognize that however many times the angels are prepared to come to our aid (and we can call on them infinitely), our way forward as a positive being, centred and sourced in the light, must be our own decision and an expression of our own will. The angels will serve, they will facilitate, they will companion, they will bear us up. But if we are in a stew of negativity, and decide not to make an effort to walk out of it along the shining path that the angels open up for us as soon as that path appears, then they can do nothing further to help us, and can only watch sadly as we enclose ourselves in our tower of darkness once again. The essential thing to remember is that humans and angels work *together*. If we think that no effort of our own is required, we actually cut ourselves off from their help. So, be a spiritual opportunist! As soon as the shining trail appears, stand upright on it. As soon as the golden door into the angelic realms takes form, grasp the handle and insist on admittance. We will grow to immediately recognize that moment, that beautiful piercing of the prevailing negativity, as we continue to work with the angels. Our own heart instantly feels the release of pressure, of oppression. In this way, we ground the angels' work into our earthly conditions.

The Sword of Michael

Archangel Michael rules the angelic hierarchy. We will learn more about his feminine consort as we progress into the new age, for her energies and consciousness are as vividly present as his in the androgynous being we know as Michael.

When you feel that a murkiness exists in the atmosphere around you, and especially when you feel negative, energy-draining attachments present in your aura or clinging to the area of your chakras, call on Archangel Michael to deliver you by means of his magical sword. (Chakras are spiritual energy-points aligned with the spine and associated with the ductless glands which connect us to our spiritual or light body. The main chakras occur at the base of the spine, at midpoint between the

navel and the pubis (this chakra, although associated with the
sex organs, is also linked to the spleen), at the solar plexus, at the
heart, in the hollow of the throat, upon the brow at the point
between the eyes, and at the crown. The crown chakra is a
double one, and also manifests directly above the brow chakra, at
the top of the forehead. This is our 'unicorn's horn' chakra.
(There are also important chakras at the centre of the hands and
the feet – *see* The Mysterious Vivaxis on page 12.)

When you call on Archangel Michael, enter the star of spiritual light (*see* Star Breathing on page 2), and let all your work with
him commence from its protective centre. (The star is, in one sense,
a manifestation of the mighty Archangel Michael).

The sword of Michael is electric blue and bright silver in
colour. It throws off shafts of blue-silver light, and its blade flashes
pure silver. Always use this sword with caution. See it cutting away
unwanted conditions and stagnant energy from around and within
your aura and your chakras, but let it work gently and with calm
precision, as a dedicated surgeon might work. The silver blade cuts
and frees, the flashing blue of the sword seals the sites where the
silver blade has descended and cleansed. Use these two qualities
of the sword in sequence, cutting and then sealing. When the
process is complete, thank Archangel Michael and ask for his con-
tinued protection and blessing.

Visualization practice with the sword of Michael is always
beneficial, for you will probably find that you need to call on its
impressive powers of emancipation many times throughout your
work with angel healing, both for yourself and for others.

The Violet Flame

The third great power tool for clearing and transforming oppressive energy is the famous Violet Flame. This was given to
humanity by Saint Germain, one of the ascended masters, who,
like all the masters concerned with our solar system, descends

from the spiritual realms from time to time to offer teaching and enlightenment to those who will listen. He gave the knowledge of the Violet Flame to Guy Ballard in the early 1930s, telling him that 'the use of the violet consuming flame is more valuable to… mankind than all the wealth, all the gold and all the jewels of this planet.' The great Archangel Zadkiel has described the Violet Flame as 'a giant electrode of cosmic energy'. When we invoke this energy, no negative emanation can stand in its way.

At the heart of the Violet Flame is the white fire that dwells within, and comprises the star of spiritual light, which we all carry within our being at the centre of the heart. Therefore, when we invoke the Violet Flame, it is best, as with the other exercises, to first step into the heart of the star in our imagination, and to call upon Archangel Michael for protection. We need to do this because, like moths to a flame, the violet fire actually attracts the darkness. We do not need to be dismayed by this, because all light, whether spiritual or physical, attracts the creatures that ensoul the mysterious darkness of the earth plane. One day, they will all be redeemed and gathered safely into the light, and their darkness will be no more. Until that time, we have to protect ourselves from them whenever we use a power so concentrated and dynamic as the Violet Flame.* The protection, once requested, is definite and assured, so we should not allow ourselves to feel any reluctance or inhibition in our use of the peerless and incomparable Violet Flame. Saint Germain is known as Lord of the Seventh Ray.

There are seven great rays of creation, depicted for us by the rainbow, which, through the magical effects of the liquid crystal in the atmosphere that we know as water, refracts the white light from the sun into seven different hues. The Seventh Ray is the ceremonial ray, the ray of beauty and power which facilitates the conjoinment of angels and human beings in service and cooperation, and so we work with this ray when we conjoin with the

*See Elizabeth Clare Prophet's excellent little book, Violet Flame, Summit University Press, USA, for further information.

healing angels in loving service. Saint Germain overlights our ceremonies with the healing angels, and delights in being called upon to give his inspiration and enlightenment to our efforts and aspirations. Although the masters have expressed a specific wish for us not to get too involved in focusing on their different personalities, it seems appropriate that we should know a little about the history of this mystical and fascinating figure. For now, however, Saint Germain would particularly stress the beauty and simplicity of using the Violet Flame each day, and even many times a day, as we tread the course of our lives. It is so simple and easy to do, that it would seem crazy not to avail ourselves of the opportunity! Using the Violet Flame liberates us into love, liberates us into light, so that we may enjoy the myriad configurations and manifestations in our life that these all-encompassing words embrace.

Decree of the Violet Flame

Enter the star of spiritual light, and call on Archangel Michael for protection.

Imagine that the seventh ray of the rainbow, like the mysterious light cascading from some hallowed violet jewel in the heavenly realms, is enfolding and illuminating you.

Its fiery essence permeates every cell, every atom and subatomic particle in your body; it enters into each and every body that is yours and comprises your soul.

It suffuses your emotions, your mind, your nervous system, your memory and subconscious.

Say three times (or as many times as you like, but at least three):

> I AM a being of violet fire!
>
> I AM the purity God desires!

At first you will think that nothing much has happened to you by invoking the Violet Flame. Just wait a little while, and note how you begin to feel! A high tide of radiant life-energy will sweep through you, carrying you forward into every task with a divine volition that has to be experienced to be appreciated. Remember – 'the use of the violet consuming flame is more valuable to mankind than all the wealth, all the gold and all the jewels of this planet.'

After working with these short and simple meditations, it is wise to seal your upper chakras. It takes only a few seconds. Just see a circle of light enclosing a bright silver cross ($+$), and hold this image briefly over your crown, at the top of your forehead in the middle (the unicorn's horn chakra which is connected to the crown centre), the middle of the brow (above and between the eyes), the hollow of the throat, the heart (this centre is located directly in the centre of the chest, rather than slightly to the left, which is where the physical heart resides), and the solar plexus (not truly one of the higher chakras, but it is always better to seal this sensitive and sometimes reactionary chakra).

Healing Hands

Let us contemplate our hands for a moment. We use them for almost every task we perform. From my own perspective, it is the use of the hands allied to the thinking and imaginal processes that makes writing and literature a manifest art form. From the humblest activity to the most sublime, we call on the magic in our hands.

The angels tell us that the ideation which became the living form of our created hands was forged from the deepest indwelling mystery within the heart of Divine Spirit. They are the cosmic twins, the mystical balance between the sacred masculine and feminine principles, the ongoing Sacred Marriage in action.

When we use their consecrated union for the purposes of cruelty
and all that comprises the death forces in any form, we fail to
realize with what potency and power we invoke the darkness.
Angelic intelligences fashioned our hands after their own image
according to divine will, for our fingers are truly rays. Our feet,
being our interface with the earth, were forged in harmony with
similar principles. Our hands and our feet were meant to conjoin
heaven and earth within ourselves, and so to balance the forces
of light and the forces of darkness, for in that balance is the
source of supernal light, the heavenly light that absorbs and
transforms the darkness and makes of it an increase in divine
radiance.

As we hope to show in our next book, Margaret Bailey and I
believe that this dynamic link between heaven and earth that
exists within ourselves is connected deeply to the Holy Grail,
and that the powers of the Grail will come amongst us again,
indeed are even imminent. Our first step towards receiving the
blessing of the Grail is to bless and honour our hands, in full
recognition and reverence of the divine purpose for which they
were created.

Important chakras exist within the palms of our hands, like a
bright circle in their centre. They are linked to the chakras in
the soles of our feet. These four chakras are further connected to
the intriguing mystery of what is called our 'Vivaxis'.

The Mysterious Vivaxis

The pioneering work of Frances Nixon brought to light this fas-
cinating phenomenon in the middle years of the 20th century.
She discovered, and went on to scientifically validate, the
marvel of the Vivaxis, described as our 'energy point of origin'.
By careful and meticulous research, she proved that we are con-
nected throughout life by lines of energy to our Vivaxis sphere.
Frances Nixon gave it this name from an amalgamation of the
Latin words *viva* (life) and *axis* (a central line around which a

rotating body moves), because her observations revealed that the life force of each individual rotated about this central point that is the Vivaxis.

The Vivaxis is a little sphere, the size of a foetus, which is usually formed in the last few weeks of a pregnancy, when the incoming soul has finally 'touched base' and has arrived securely in the body of the unborn baby (although it actually takes 21 years to thoroughly 'ground' the soul in the physical body, which is the inner reason why we associate our 21st birthday with 'coming of age'). At this point, the little Vivaxis sphere is released into the earth and fixes there, generally at some spot where the mother lived or spent time in the final few weeks of gestation. There it faithfully remains, however far its owner travels from the site of its location.

Frances Nixon explains that the atomic particles inside the Vivaxis energy sphere align themselves with, and become magnetized to, the geophysical field in which the Vivaxis 'earths' itself. This magnetizing of the energies causes a wave link to establish itself between the Vivaxis sphere and its owner which remains constant regardless of distance.

There is a bilateral flow of energy between ourselves and our Vivaxis. The energy flow coming to us from the Vivaxis travels vertically until it reaches our current altitude, then horizontally until it reaches our left foot, switching to a vertical flow once again as it moves up our left leg to our left hand. The flow of energy returns to the Vivaxis sphere in a vertical direction through our right foot up to our right hand, wherefrom it flows in an outgoing horizontal direction from our right hand.

There is good reason to believe (*see* my book, *Your Guardian Angel*) that the Vivaxis is actually our eighth or our earth chakra, expressed through our hands and our feet. Our eighth chakra is magenta in colour, a combination of red and violet, for our first chakra at the base of our spine is associated with the first ray of the rainbow, whose colour is red, and with the last ray of the rainbow, whose colour is violet. These make an octave, an harmonic, a complete sphere of creation. The rainbow (the half circle) shows us the seven rays, but if we pick up a compact disk (the full circle) and look into its mirroring surface, we will see the seven colours of the rainbow plus the hue of the earth chakra, the eighth chakra, depicted in glorious magenta. This most holy eighth chakra is the one that connects heaven and earth within our very being. Its signature is wholeness, is healing. We can draw on its strength, its wisdom and its potency by consciously developing the sleeping chakras in our hands.

We can help to activate and to purify this eighth chakra of the hands and the feet by consciously connecting with our Vivaxis. Just think of the little sphere of your Vivaxis, the same size as you were when in your foetal stage, so precious because it declares, beyond contradiction, that you contain the earth within yourself, that you are the octave which is the vibration of the earth sphere; and, therefore, you hold the destiny and the future of the earth in your hands.

First, it is a good idea to locate our Vivaxis, because by this means we can visualize the heaven and earth forces flowing through it and circulating through our hands much more easily.

Locating the Vivaxis

Take two pendulums, or objects on a chain. Hold one chain in each hand.

Stand erect, with feet apart, your heels touching (so that a V shape is created between your feet).

Gently turn clockwise, a few degrees at a time.

Note the motion of the chains in your hand. When they swing back and forth in alternating movements, you are aligned with your Vivaxis. (If the chains swing in unison, you are standing at right angles to it.)

Once you have aligned your body with your Vivaxis, you can carry out the following exercise:

Stand quietly, without holding either pendulum, and begin to be aware that you are receiving a flow of energy from your Vivaxis.

It is coming in beneath your left foot, travelling up your left leg, and entering your left hand. Just feel this for a moment or two.

Now sense the Vivaxis energy crossing the trunk of your body between the solar plexus and the sacral chakras.

As it does so, the energy connects with your navel, and then carries on down the inside of your right leg until it enters your right foot.

From there, it climbs the outside of your right leg until it enters your right hand.

It is at this point that the energy flows back to your Vivaxis: the outgoing energy becomes the returning flow as it enters the right foot and travels back up the right leg to the right hand, at which point it actually leaves the body.

When you have a clear sense of the direction and the circulation of the Vivaxis energy, open your right hand, slightly cupping the palm, and call on your guardian angel. Ask it to oversee this exercise.

Using your breath, drawing it through your heart, and using the clear visualization of the star in the heart, send bright white starlight, of a beautiful, pristine, coruscating purity, out with the Vivaxis energy leaving your right hand.

Say to your own guardian angel: 'Guardian angel,

please bring all safely into balance and harmony;
please circulate the white light seven times throughout me and my Vivaxis. Please bless, protect and
stabilize my earth chakra.'

Visualize the beautiful white starlight coming back
into your left foot with the Vivaxis energy; and then
watch it flow in and out, to complete the circuit seven
times.

Ask for the blessing of Divine Mother and her angels
on your earth chakra.

Thank your guardian angel for its help.

Attune to the chakras in your hands, and see them as agents of
blessing that can heal and transform. In all your work in healing
with angels, you will use your hands in some capacity either
humble or sublime. We need often to wash our hands in spiritual
substance so that their energies do not become jaded. We can do
this by using the following simple exercises.

Starlight Hand-Bathing

Become aware of the gentle spiritual light emanating
from your heart-centre.

Look into the star shining peacefully there with your
soul vision, and imagine a pearly white candle in your
left hand.

Place it within the star in your heart, and see it take
flame.

Lift it out again with your right hand and place it in
front of you.

Watch this pearly candle for a moment as it burns with
a white-golden flame.

Wash your hands thoroughly in the flame (it is quite painless!), and feel the invigorating purity of the spiritual starlight cleansing and blessing your hands until their chakras shine like the sun.

Angel of the Chaste Hands

Call on the female angel Ouestucati (Oo-stu-cahti) to wash away all impurities from your hands. Ouestucati is a beautiful female angel, known as 'the lady of the chaste hands'. She will perform this important task for you if you do not happen to have the few moments necessary to carry out the ceremony above. Just hold out your hands to Ouestucati and slowly turn them around as if washing them as you call on her and receive her ministrations.

Of course, you can combine both ceremonies for a power-cleanse! It is very important to look after the spiritual hygiene of your hands, both before and after healing ceremonies, especially if your hands come in contact with someone who is suffering pain, sickness, mental disturbance or depression. In each case, the cleansing power of water is also necessary.

Remember always that your hands are mystic symbols of the highest potency, and that they were fashioned by angels, according to the law of Divine Spirit, in their own miraculous image.

Absorbing the Love of the Angels

Before beginning this programme of angel healing, just sit quietly for a minute or two and absorb the love of the angels. Their love is perfect, free from all taints, and they always celebrate the highest and the best in us. The darkness, the faults and the foolhardiness that exist in our makeup they enfold in compassion and tenderly seek to unlock the chains that bind us. No matter how shamefully petty and unworthy our thoughts and actions have been, we can confide in our angel friends and be assured of no judgement or reproach. They will offer us only profound understanding and kindness, and shine a light onto a way out of any confusion or distress we may feel.

But it is not only when in confusion or distress that we turn to the love of the angels. It is not something we should feel duty-bound to do because we want to advance our spirituality or learn angel healing techniques or cleanse ourselves from negativity. It is simply a joy, a treat, some special time for ourselves during which nothing is required of us except that we should relax and feel good: soothed and stilled and comforted at the deepest levels. Accept the angels' gift of love. It is a gift of happiness that they offer perpetually and unstintingly as an expression of their grace, their abundance and their delight in giving.

The Angel of the Pointing Hand

We return to our contemplation of this angel, who urges us to look to and aspire to the highest in our angel communion and healing, and indeed in all things. Who is the angel of the pointing hand?; this mysterious teacher who, in his burning intensity, may seem a little stern, but who is yet all compassion, all love. He sounds a clarion call to our soul, to our deepest indwelling spirit, and that is why he seems to some to be a little intimidating, for he stirs our awareness of our more profound self, with all it majestic potentialities and fabulous hidden treasure.

We may associate the angel of the pointing hand with that circle of angels who are known as the 'Ancient of Days'. These are 'the holy ones of the highest', the most exalted among the angel clan. The Ancient of Days has been cited by the first teachers of angel lore as 'both the Eternity and the Time of all things prior to days and eternity and time'. In other words, this angel, or circle of angels, encompasses the emanations of Divine Spirit, and was in existence before material, measurable, linear time began.

They are headed by Macroposopus, 'vast countenance', who is of the ineffable living essence of God. We can appreciate, therefore, that our angel of the pointing hand is indeed in earnest about directing our aspirations, our consciousness, to the 'highest of the high'! He manifests as a being of white light of measureless purity. But if we are overawed by his sternness and gravity, we can reflect that through him shines the peerless Michael, friend and comforter of stumbling humankind, and that Michael himself emanates the all-enfolding love of the Shekinah, the Feminine Shining One, who dispenses her blessing with unequalled tenderness and sanctity. Through her kindly benediction, those highest heights do not appal or daunt us; we know that they are not unattainable or far away, but here within the mystery of our hearts, and that we can find them in simplicity, in peace, as we quietly walk the earth.

CHAPTER TWO

HOW TO CONTACT THE HEALING ANGELS

The Seven Tools of Communion

There are seven tools of communion with which we can contact the angels. Other systems and cultures will no doubt be able to enlarge upon these, but I have always found the following spiritual implements more than adequate for contacting the angels:

- the breath
- meditation (including prayer and invocation)
- the silence
- imagination
- the heart
- the chakras
- ceremony

The Breath

The Angel of the Holy Breath is one of the great healing angels. When working with her, I have found that the sense of her presence grows almost tangible, and that awareness of her might and majesty is simultaneous with a beautiful reassurance that she tenderly sustains and enfolds us within her protective, life-giving aura. If you are feeling disconnected from your source, just sit quietly and ask the Angel of the Holy Breath to breathe with you. This can be a deeply calming and grounding experience, and can lift you high into the angelic realms.

Spiritual teachers assure us that our breath is magical. The angels infuse us with their essence, enter into us and commune with us, through the medium of air – our breath. The breath plays a crucial part in opening the door to the spiritual worlds. We cannot attune to our soul without the aid of the breath and we cannot release ourselves from the grip of the earthly planes without attuning to the soul. Our soul ascends on our breath, lit from within by the radiance of our spirit. The act of magical breathing and attunement to the soul must be carried out via the heart-centre. We have to breathe 'through the heart', inhaling and exhaling through this chakra, because the breath is our yoke to Goddess-God.

It will seem very natural to draw in the breath and release it in this way. When we breathe 'through the heart', we are breathing in the brilliant light of the Godhead which fills our being. We can then direct this ineffable light to the world, to humanity, to the troubled heart of another, to any negative condition which needs healing. As long as it is given as a free gift from the heart, the breath will sustain this pure light which shines from the spirit through the soul. Judgement and opinions must not be allowed to intrude, for they carry the contamination of the ego, which disconnects us from the ineffable source of Divine Spirit.

A beautiful way to attune to the magic of the breath is to use the Star Breathing technique described in the first exercise of Chapter One. Indeed, we cannot commence magical, focused breathing without lighting the mystical star in the heart. Our breath, our quiet inward focus, are the natural lighteners of this exquisite indwelling star.

There exists a method of breathing called 'the Mother's Breath' which is based on the seven and one or the octave rhythm, the Law of Eight, which we explored in the previous chapter in relation to the seven traditional chakras and the eighth or earth chakra that operates through our hands and feet. This is an excellent meditational focus for the breath, and its mystical rhythm will assist and bless our attunement to the great healing angels. It signifies the seven rays or principles of creation held within the mystery of the All – the seven and the one. It will, in particular, help you to contact and breathe in harmony with the Angel of the Holy Breath, although your communion with this great angel should always be simple and natural, and without formal structure of any kind if that is how you prefer to work with her. Nevertheless, practising the method of 'the Mother's Breath' until you feel comfortable with it will yield wonderful results. It is very easy to follow.

The Mother's Breath

Breathe in to a count of seven.

Pause and hold the breath for one count.

Breathe out to the count of seven.

Pause again for one count.

Breathe in to the count of seven and resume the cycle.

Avoid forcing the rhythm or allowing yourself to become breathless or uncomfortable in any way. Be as brief or as long as you wish concerning the length of time you take to count out the seven beats for the in-breath, the seven for the out-breath and the length of time you take for the pauses in between. Let comfort and ease be your guiding factors, and take care not to jerk the breath as you count to seven. Let your breathing be smooth and relaxed in its rise and fall, and let the prompt of your counting come as if from a distance, hardly noticed except to subtly and unobtrusively measure out the rhythm.

We need to practise this art of magical breathing each day, whether we perform all the exercises given or just choose to sit quietly and simply focus on our breathing and find our own rhythm, because it is an essential component of healing with the angels. We give and receive perpetually through our breath.

There is a little meditational exercise we can do if we are feeling tired and depleted after giving healing, or if we are in need ourselves. It concerns the fairylike enchantment of the northern lights. The miracle of this natural phenomenon may seem unconnected with the act of breathing, but in fact it is the angels of the air, and so the angels of the breath, who long to bear us up into the mysteries of the Aurora Borealis. Philip Pullman, in his trilogy *His Dark Materials*, has written an inspired account of a city existing within the northern lights. This is indeed true, although it is not a city which exists on the material plane, thus reflecting earthly cities, but a citadel of wonder and spiritual delight pulsating far above the mundane sphere.

Two versions of the exercise are given. In Meditation 1, we can absorb the beautiful emerald light that the Aurora Borealis often displays as a vast green heavenly lake, a single hue which is a manifestation of the sacred green ray, the ray of the heart. In this meditation, we contain and conserve our energies, resting in deep peace within the great heart of creation. This soothes and revivifies our heart-centre.

The Northern Lights (Meditation 1)

Enter a light meditation, using one of the breathing techniques specified above.

Let the angels of the air surround you, and take you up into the starlit night towards the holy north.

There you see before you the enchantment of the dancing northern lights, huge sheets of lustrous fire appearing and reappearing in a dreamlike ecstasy of motion.

The angels bear you right into the centre of the aery magical dance.

Now you are a winged being, as they are, and you are swept into the heart of their balletic mystery.

Bathe in the colour of the dance, the colour of the Aurora Borealis, which is deep, emerald green, swathes of sacred green, the green of the spirit of the earth...

When you are ready, allow the angels of the air to gently bear you back down to earth.

Seal your chakras, and, because the northern lights are imbued with fairy magic, stamp your feet (very gently, or you will shock your centres) three times!

In Meditation 2, we visualize the Aurora Borealis as it manifests in many colours, allowing the soul to delight in their coruscating, effervescent vitality and to become a vehicle for the expression and play of their forces. This energizes and stimulates our crown centre.

The Northern Lights (Meditation 2)

Enter a light meditation, using one of the breathing techniques specified above.

Let the angels of the air surround you, and take you up into the starlit night towards the holy north.

There you see before you the enchantment of the dancing northern lights, huge sheets of lustrous fire appearing and reappearing in a dreamlike ecstasy of motion.

The angels bear you right into the centre of the aery magical dance.

Now you are a winged being, as they are, and you are swept into the heart of their balletic mystery.

Bathe in the colours of the dance, the fairy hues of the northern lights, teeming in every tint of the rainbow and more. Let this many-coloured garment swirl over you and carry you into the secret soul of the being who is the Aurora Borealis...

When you are ready, allow the angels of the air to gently bear you back down to earth.

Seal your chakras, and, because the northern lights are imbued with fairy magic, stamp your feet (very gently, or you will shock your centres) three times!

You will be surprised how energized and revitalized you feel after these breathing meditations. Angels informed Geoffrey Hodson, the angel seer, that there are vast magnetic energies locked up within the air, huge reservoirs and streams of magnetic force that embody an awe-inspiring life and consciousness we have yet to understand. 'Great electric roads through space exist,' the angels told him, 'pathways through the atmosphere created by currents of electric force.' These majestic highways do not exist randomly, and their appearance does not only denote climatic phenom-ena. One day, the angels promise us, we will walk these grand highways of the soul with fireshod feet. Until we can do this in full consciousness, we can enjoy their revivifying effects on both our nervous system and our subtle bodies in meditation.

When the northern lights are at play, fairy and angelic soul-presence and energy are abroad, and there is every reason to take imaginal advantage of their manifestation!

Meditation (Including Prayer and Invocation)

The Angel of Meditation is Iahhel (I-ah-hel). We can call on this great angelic luminary for help in undertaking our medita-tions. From her flow great streams of inner peace, illumination, and the angel magic that unlocks inner doors and guarded entryways.

We cannot properly advance into higher consciousness unless we meditate. In seeking the supernal worlds, we need to under-stand that their essence, their keynote, their vibration, is that of love. Therefore, we prepare ourselves for meditation by quietly opening our being to universal love.

There is a life deep within our being which is far more vital, significant and beautiful than the mundane level at which we normally operate. It is this point of peace we need to seek. It is enshrined in our heart-centre and will lead us through into the inner spheres.

We find the doorway into meditation by focusing gently on the breath. Sitting in a quiet place, spine erect and supported if necessary, place your right ankle lightly over your left (this seals your energy field) and cup your left hand in your right. Centre your awareness on your breathing, imagining that you are drawing in and giving out each cycle of breath through the heart.

Now think of the highest plane of which you can conceive, and give this sphere an image. It might be the Christ, the Goddess, Buddha, Krishna, Divine Mother, Brigid (goddess of the Celts), Mary (Magdalene or Mother Mary), or one of the archangels. It might be a bright candle flame, or a golden point in the centre of a circle of light, or a jewel pulsating softly with perfect light. Whatever brings you into the beauty and the peace of the Divine Presence will lead you to and through the doorway that opens onto the higher worlds.

Rest your awareness in your heart-centre, gazing upon the image in your mind's eye, and open your heart to love. If you feel resistance or anger, or simply cannot feel anything very much, see a single pink rose in your heart opening to the golden sunlight and giving forth its heavenly fragrance. Inhale the perfume and, if you choose, softly begin to chant the word 'Ham' as you breathe in, and 'Sah' as you exhale. In ancient Sanskrit, *Ham* means 'I Am' and *Sah* means 'Divine Spirit' or 'Divine Spark'. This will help you to contact the healing source of love in your being.

When intruding thoughts assault your meditation, just return all your attention as an act of conscious will, yet with great respect and gentleness, to focus once more on the sanctuary of your heart, the steady rhythm of your breathing and chanting, and your chosen image. If your intrusive thoughts become very disturbing and clamorous, offer them to the Being upon whom you are meditating, or, if your chosen image is other than a personification, give the distracting thoughts into the care of the Lord or Mistress of your Temple (your higher self). If your mind starts to drift into cogitation and you have difficulty controlling it, it can be helpful to say very firmly out loud, 'I choose to meditate. I choose Silence.' Then return to the elements of your meditation as described above. Gradually you will come to a place of utter peace and calm, beyond and beneath the busy traffic of your thought processes. When this occurs you have found the point of entry, and will pass through into the worlds within.

If even a split second of vision or breakthrough to a higher plane is beyond your reach at first, refuse the temptation to abandon meditation in disgust or despair! Your breakthrough will indeed come, the door will open before too long. This is incontrovertible cosmic law. It is just a matter of persistence in your practice of meditation.

When you are ready to finish your meditation, it is essential to protect your finer vehicles, your non-physical bodies, by sealing your chakras, to which they are connected. The seven main 'star gates' or chakras are located at the crown, mid-brow between the eyes, the hollow of the throat, the heart (the chakra point is located more to the centre of the chest than is the physical heart), the solar plexus, just below the navel, and the base of the spine, situated above the anus.

Imagine a ring of light surrounding an equal-sided cross of bright silver, and seal each of your centres with this powerful protective symbol (just place it in imagination over each chakra). If you still feel vulnerable or dreamy, imagine a spiral of light emerging from under your left foot and making seven golden clockwise spiralling rings around you from your feet to above your crown. Then see the head of the spiral run straight down the line of your chakras like a rod of light from your crown to the ground below your feet. Never forget to complete at least the sealing exercise, or you will lose the benefit of your meditation. If your meditation has been short and simple, it is only necessary to seal the first four chakras.

If you ever find it difficult to commence meditation (sometimes the pressures of the outer world are all too present), imagine a golden pyramid towering before you. Seven wide stairs lead to its pinnacle. Climb these stairs to the top of the golden pyramid, and begin your meditation from there.

The power and felicity of prayer and invocation cannot be underestimated and are indispensable, especially in the field of angel healing. Later, we will learn to invoke Raphael and the healing angels, and the angels of mercy. For the purposes of healing, it is also necessary to find our own angelic name (*see* page 80) – that part of us which resonates with the angelic kingdom and which might be thought of as 'the angel within'. Prayers to offer to the healing angels are given throughout this book. For general prayers and invocations to the angels, see my books, *Summoning Angels* and *Your Guardian Angel*.

The Silence

The angels have told us that there is a mighty power in silence. Harpocratos is one of the names of the hushed, enfolding Angel of Silence. The silence, and the ensouling Angel of the Silence, bequeaths to us the power to still our mind and our emotions, without which we cannot contact the healing angels. Silence was a goddess of the ancient world, a spiritual being embodying the dimensions of a principle. We might say that silence is a quality endowed with goddess-force. It is a worthwhile endeavour to intone a prayer to Silence herself, asking her to enfold us in her presence.

Having prayed to absorb silence, and to be absorbed into the silence, see the orb of the full moon sailing in silver peace in a midnight-blue sky. It is Silence herself, hanging in hushed calm above you.

See a flight of seven crystal stairs spiralling upwards from the earth to the gates of the moon, which shine like pearl. Mount the steps and walk through the pearly arch of the open gates. Feel the silence take you into itself, utterly enclosing you in another world – the world of silence.

The silence is the higher aspect of your soul. Seek it every day, if only for a few moments. Your breath leads you into silence as you practise the imagery, and sustains you there. Listen, and you will hear the Breath of the silence.

Imagination

The Angel of the Imagination is the bright angel Samandiriel (Sam-an diri-el). We can call on the evocative consciousness of this shining one to unlock the spiritual power of our imagination.

Imagination has been spoken of by the ascended masters as the divine faculty connecting us to truth. When the Old Testament gave us the revelation that we are made in God's image, it intimated that we were given the creative power of the Godhead as a special grace. That creative principle is the imagination. It dwells within us as a living potential of unconscionable magnitude. Everything that comes into being has to be *imagined* first, even the simplest, humblest things. Learn to trust and to revere your imagination. It is the golden key to the spiritual worlds.

Imagination is our divine gift – a window on truth – a tool for inner sight. When the imagination and the intuition work hand in hand, you will truly be able to walk with angels. They are almost the same faculty. Imagination is the clarity of seeing, intuition is the wisdom of knowing. Whilst Samandiriel is the angel who presides over and blesses the imagination, Brigid is the goddess who succours the imagination and the intuition, in her role as mistress of creative fire and the crystal clarity of the soul. Always there are the two aspects feeding us in life – the angelic life-stream on the one hand, and the human on the other.

If you have difficulty in using your imagination, or faculty of creative visualization, begin by endeavouring to see in your mind's eye some simple objects, such as different fruits. Imagine a bright yellow banana, a shiny red apple, a golden pear, a round, smooth hazelnut. Picture them one by one as vividly as you can, and hold them in mental focus for as long as is comfortable. Then repeat the exercise; only this time, as you create them in your imagination, also create their taste on your tongue. Make them delicious – the very best banana, apple, pear and hazel nut, et cetera, that you have ever tasted. Soon, your imagination, with all its subtle inner senses, will begin to awaken within you, and you will be thrilled by the new worlds that will begin to open up to you.

Here are some images to help you imagine your imagination! See your imagination as:

- A shining mirror
- A magic casement onto fairy worlds
- A crystal bowl filled with well-water of a miraculous purity and clarity
- A candle of vision, lit and softly shining
- A velvet curtain being drawn back upon a window onto a magnificent starry night
- A flight-craft
- An ancient entryway into a vast circular cavern filled with jewels and marvellous treasure
- A deep, pure well with a single star glimmering mystically in its waters
- A great, carved door, overhung with ivy tendrils and flowers, opening slowly onto luminous lands of the soul
- A bright white unicorn who steals softly to your side, and nudges you to mount and ride away under the moon to the high places which call to your soul
- The Grail castle, supernaturally present in a moonlit and starlit glade, upon which you have come after journeying through dark forests. Its door stands open, and festive lights and sounds of a noble company glance and float like enchantment from within
- A silver stairway to the moon
- A rainbow bridge, iridescent with soft spiritual fire, leading into the realms of the angels

- An enchanted fairy isle, to which you set sail in a boat with silver sails and a living swan at its prow
- A monumental clear quartz crystal in a circular white temple, into whose heart-depths you step as easily as if you passed into a ray of starlight
- Follow a peal of bells that sound upon a wild and lovely sea shore, until you walk into the sparkling blue sea and descend rapturously to the mythical Country-under-Wave, more full of marvels than your deepest dreams
- An open book in an ancient monastic scriptorium, over which you are poised with feathered pen and luminous inks filled with jewelled light, full of wonder and awe at the thought of what you will bring to life upon the waiting leaves of virgin vellum
- An exquisitely carved key, wrought by elven hands and angel magic, which unlocks the mystery of your heart

Conjuring several of these dreamlike inscapes should help you to begin to understand what your imagination truly is, and to tread its supernatural starlit highway with due reverence and wonder.

The healing angels tell us that the heart-centred imagination is the golden key to unlocking the door through which they flock to help us in our times of need and crisis. To make full use of their gifts, we must honour their wisdom, and embrace our imagination wholeheartedly. We have been programmed to disdain and generally 'dis' the faculty of our imagination. Let us triumphantly reclaim it, and take our power back!

The Heart

Wisdom teaching associates the heart with the sun, for the heart is indeed the sun, the centre of the cosmos of our being, around which our physical life and, in truth, our spiritual consciousness, revolves or circulates. Francis Thompson, an English poet writing in the early years of the 20th century, gives a teaching on the consciousness of the heart in one of his most famous poems:

Where is the land of Luthany,

Where is the tract of Elenore?

I am bound therefor.

'Pierce thy heart to find the key;

With thee take

Only what none else would keep:

Learn to dream when thou dost wake,

Learn to wake when thou dost sleep…

When thy seeing blindeth thee

When their sight to thee is sightless;

Their living, death; their light, most lightless!

Search no more –

Pass the gates of Luthany, tread the region Elenore.'

Where is the land of Luthany,

And where the region Elenore?

I do faint therefor.

'When to the new eyes of thee

All things by immortal power

Near or far,

Hiddenly

To each other link-ed are,

That thou canst not stir a flower

Without troubling of a star;

    Seek no more,

O seek no more!

Pass the gates of Luthany, tread the region Elenore.'

From 'The Mistress of Vision'

These are the words of an angel speaking to a pilgrim, a seeker on the path. The land of Luthany is that higher vision, that awakened state, which the pilgrim or the seeker (the striving soul) longs to attain, so that the gates might open into the spiritual worlds. The enlightenment the soul seeks is 'the land of Luthany', the world of the spirit 'the region Elenore'. The angel gives to the pilgrim a beautiful mystery teaching so that s/he may at last 'pass the gates of Luthany, tread the region Elenore'.

We see that the angel bids the pilgrim 'pierce thy heart to find the key'. In the ancient mystery schools, the neophyte was taught that heart-consciousness, the mind in the heart, was the great key to the mystery of all creation and of approach to the Godhead itself. This heart-consciousness is not the seat of the emotions and of nervous or instinctual energy (which actually lies in the solar plexus) but is the source of the power of love, which is divine. It may be difficult to think of love as a power, rather than an emotion, in essence, because we experience love through our emotions. Nevertheless, experiencing love through the medium of our emotions does not mean that love itself is an emotion. Love is the sacred flame arising from the Source of All. It may help to think of the power of a storm in its crescendo – terrible, ineluctable – and yet at the heart of this mighty play of forces there is a profound and perfect stillness. Manifest creation and the moods and passions which inform it are the storm, love is the mystical peace at its heart.

The mystery schools taught that at the heart of all created things, all created beings, there is a spark of the holy light of the Godhead. In human beings, that spark is bestowed in a special way, bearing with it a stupendous gift; for through it, we as individuals are given the opportunity to grow into God-Goddess-consciousness.

The great symbol and sign of the Divine Being for humankind has always been the sun. We are told that there is a huge central sun, the heart of the cosmos, around which all the lesser suns in the universe move, and that every sun or star bears within its physical form the perfect shape of a six-pointed star which emanates the white and golden spiritual light shining behind the atoms of material sunlight. The golden-white light of the star is love-in-action and pours forth from the Godhead which is its ineffable origin. It is a spark of this sacred light which quickens every being, and which links the human heart directly to the sun and the Divine Being, of which our sun is but a flicker of manifestation. The sun of the human body is the heart, and the heart it is which enshrines that mysterious spark of Godhead which when nurtured by our own striving rises as a column of flame so that the head-centre gives off a halo of light like the physical sun. Nevertheless, the root and the source of this flame is in the heart, not the head or the mind.

The flame or spark in the heart is also a star, a tiny micro-cosm of the macrocosmic six-pointed star which exists at the centre of every heavenly body in the cosmos. This golden-white star exists within our own heart, in actuality, in reality. It is the source of all our power, all our creativity. By its grace, we give and receive healing and spiritual illumination. To this great in-breath and out-breath of spiritual life the angels tend and minister.

This profound teaching is given by the angel to the pilgrim in Francis Thompson's poem. The angels of the sun, of love, says the angel, will come to us to 'pierce our hearts' when we aspire to rise into the reality of the spirit. When we can renounce earthly values and illusions ('With thee take only what none else would keep'), when we can stimulate our inner vision ('Learn to dream when thou dost wake, Learn to wake when thou dost sleep...') and realize our unity with all creation, our brotherhood with all beings ('That thou canst not stir a flower without troubling of a star'), the key will turn in the sacred lock, and the door will open onto the region Elenore – the worlds within: the realm of the heart, the innermost chamber of the spiritual sun, which is where the angels dwell.

Michael and Shekinah are the two great Shining Ones who rule the sun. Servants of these mighty angels who are also con-nected with the sun (amongst countless others) are Anael, the Angel of the Star of Love, Jophiel ('Beauty of God') and Raziel, Lord of the Supreme Mysteries. They will bless all our healing endeavours when we work from heart-centred awareness.

The Chakras

Our seven main chakras are the points of connection of our physical body to the structure and spiritual vivification of the inner worlds of Divine Spirit. They can become vulnerable, polluted, and under- or overcharged. We have to learn how to seal, balance and cleanse them.

The chakras will be dealt with more fully in a later chapter. For now, it will be helpful to your healing endeavours to visualize the chakras as a stairway to heaven, consisting of seven great golden steps, each one guarded by an angel. Climb these steps to the eighth level, which looks out onto a night of softly glimmering stars.

These are the stars of our universe, but they are also luminous points of spiritual potential to which we are subtly connected. The vision of Jacob's ladder is connected to the design of our chakra system and its inherent magic.

Mary Magdalene is the great mistress of the chakra system, which is known as the 'Seven Virgins of Light'. Call on her to cleanse, bless and inspire each of your chakras, and to teach you their profound mysteries.

Ceremony

Simple ceremony, conducted in a prepared purity of mind, atmosphere and environment, is the prescription of the angels for our healing endeavours. Elaborate ceremony throughout many cultures has been the keynote of the past, and whilst such complex ceremony is undoubtedly very powerful, it has often been corrupted, or distorted into shadowy channels. When ceremony is simple and conducted from the heart, it retains its great power, but does not steer a course that runs close to the encroachment of darkness, because the mind and the mental bodies of the healing practitioner are not tempted into the fascination of unbalanced complexity. (The ascended spiritual teacher White Eagle has advised us that our brain, as much as any other bodily organ, can become seized by a sense of its own power and domination, and begin to indulge in self-gratification.)

As we progress into the Aquarian age, we will find that we as individuals, and the civilizations we comprise, begin to respond more and more to the seventh ray of creation, the ceremonial ray. This ray is violet (the ceremony of the Violet Flame (*see* Chapter One) is intimately associated with it), and is also known as the Ray of Beauty.

The healing angels tell us that, as their human co-workers, our great triple task is to educate, to cleanse, and to attune. We perform all three under the influence of the seventh ray, although of course there is no limitation, and all the gifts of the seven great rays will be involved to some degree in our healing work. A simple herbal correspondence with the seventh ray consists of violet and lavender flowers, used for purification throughout the centuries (the name lavender is associated with the French *laver*, meaning to wash). We will see how such simple inclusions as these humble flowers in our healing rituals can tap a vast reservoir of therapeutic and restorative power, administered and dispensed by the healing angels.

All of the healing rituals in this book are simple, and, I hope, easily memorized. The balance of simplicity, and ease and clarity of thought, are essential in our angel healing ceremonies as we come under the influence of the seventh ray. The use of ceremonial power is in itself a characteristic of the seventh ray. Another is our urge to seek and employ unseen forces and intelligences in our projects, endeavours and spiritual missions on earth. As we see, healing with the angels fully expresses these two majestic, innovative and dynamic qualities of the seventh ray. A sense of power and adventure can arise from exploring these principles, which is good; but it must be balanced by a keen sense of humility, simplicity and an inner attunement, a ready obedience, to the dictates of our higher nature, or we may find ourselves thoroughly scuppered!

One of the ancient civilizations who profoundly understood the significance of simple but deeply beautiful, evocative, and powerful ceremony was that of the Native Americans. They were not nomadic during the greatest days of their empire, although they always lived close to nature. The angels told Geoffrey Hodson: 'Those who would find us must learn to contact Nature far more intimately than is at present possible to the average man. In addition to a deeper appreciation of the beauty of Nature there must be that reverence for all her forms and moods, for all her manifold expression, which springs from a recognition of the presence of the Divine of which these forms, moods, and beauties are but the outward expression.' The Native American tribes understood this angel wisdom, and their way of life resonated with it.

The following guided visualization takes us into the heart of the famous medicine wheel of the Native Americans, a gift of manifestation and of knowledge that was bestowed directly on the tribes by the 'Shining Spirits', or the angels. When giving these guided visualizations in my workshops, we start with the 'contemplation' in preparation for the material that is to follow, which is also offered here.

Contemplation

The wisdom and philosophy of the Native Americans is at last beginning to be perceived in all its mystery, beauty and majesty. It is believed that their civilization is much older than conventionally perceived, and through their legends runs a golden thread of revelation. The spiritual teacher White Eagle speaks of a heritage of folk-tales and myths among the tribes which tell of the coming of the 'feathered Gods', people who came from afar bringing a radiance and a salvation which the American Indians wove into the fabric of their philosophy and religion.

In her book, *Sun Men of the Americas*, Grace Cooke tells of L Taylor Hansen's personal encounters with Native Americans who told him their stories of a saint or a prophet who sailed to their lands, often called 'Heah-Wah-Sah' ('he from afar off'). Each legend portrays him very similarly. He is described as beautiful, radiant, with fair complexion, fair hair and blue eyes, and he wore a white robe with exquisite embroidery of the cross round its edges. He healed the sick, spoke wisdom and brought the dead to life. L Taylor Hansen quotes from one of the elders, an old and venerated Indian, who tells the 'Legend of the Sacred City':

> ...Tonight I am here to take you walking back through the dawn-star cycles to a time long distant when the land was not as you see it.
>
> Past the memories of our grandfathers' grandfathers I take you with me to the days of the Healer, and the

times of our people's greatness…Coming north from our
Capital City, where the Mississippi meets the Missouri,
in the long-boats of the traders, the Prophet made his
journey towards the city we called Sacred…This city
was called Sacred because it was in the centre of the
Cross of Waters from whence ran the rivers to the Four
Oceans. East to the sunrise ran the waters, and north-
wards to the Sea of Dancing Lights; to the west beyond
the Great Divide the waters ran to the Sea of the
Sunset, while the Missouri and the Mississippi ran to
the Southern Sea, the Sea of the Karibs.

To this, the City of the Great Cross of Waters, up the
river called the Father of Waters, one golden morning
came the Healer. The dawn cascaded down upon him
as he left the ships of the merchants, painting his hair
and beard with beauty and lighting up his lofty features.
The streets were petalled with flowers before him as he
walked towards the Temple. Greatly beloved now was
the Pale-God, known as the Lord of Wind and Water.
His every move bespoke his kindness, his very touch
revealed his divinity and before him bowed down all
people.

Through rows of temple worshippers he moved in quiet
solemnity, holding up his hand in blessing, that hand
with the strange palm marking, for through it was
engraved the cross which he had taken as his symbol.
There at the temple he abode among us though he
often rode away with the merchants or more often
walked to distant villages, holding in his hand his great
staff, and stopping to speak with all, from the aged to
the children.

Further legends in L Taylor Hansen's book, *He Walked the Americas*, tell how Heah-Wah-Sah came down from Venus, instructing his Indian brethren to look to the star as a holy symbol for their prayers and spiritual inspiration, and how he taught them to resolve their problems by counselling together in peace.

White Eagle says in *Sun Men of the Americas*:

> The story is that Heah-Wah-Sah came mysteriously to the Indian peoples and taught them about the wonderful life beyond the sun; taught them the lessons of peace, brotherhood and goodwill, and all the beautiful truths which Jesus the Christ also taught all his disciples. At the appointed time the Indians saw him depart. He is supposed to have entered his canoe and sailed away down the river to the west, right into the sun. His symbol was that of the all-seeing eye.

> Try to forget all you have read and heard about savage Indians living in wigwams. Not all Indians were nomadic. The Indians of whom we speak had beautiful buildings, beautiful homes. In spite of all the misrepresentations our ancient Indian brethren were simple at heart – so simple and loving and gentle. They were men and women of character and strength of purpose, possessing great courage and endurance. There were many tribes, they spoke many languages, and lived at many different levels of development, but one factor all had in common, and this was a deep sense of honour and morality, of goodness. The Indian culture goes back far beyond any known historical or archaeological records of the ancient Red Indian civilization.

> It is very little understood by the present-day scholar, and it cannot easily be interpreted because man has not developed that spiritual quality which will enable him to read the truth found on the stone tablets and remnants of earlier civilizations buried in the distant

forests, not only in South America and Mexico, but in North America too. The civilization of the Indian was one of the most beautiful and ancient civilizations there has ever been on earth.

The symbol of the Indian peace-pipe is an enduring one. May we ever inhale the spirit, give it out and share it in cycles of loving peace.

The Starlit Canyon

Begin to draw your breath gently 'through the heart', envisioning this centre in your creative imagination as a sacred crystal of many facets, bearing six points which cast rays of wondrous living brightness in every direction. Dwell quietly at the midpoint of this star-crystal, for it is your true self and its facets are aspects of your soul-temple through which the eternal flame of your spirit shines.

You are drifting in the night sky among the stars. You float very slowly, very gently, as if you were becalmed in an invisible boat. All around you is the quiet darkness and the soft glistening of the stars, twinkling like genii-treasure in a vast hidden cave.

One exquisite star shines purer and clearer than the rest. As you enjoy its bright crystalline radiance which falls over you with a faery grace, the knowledge comes to you that this celestial body is not a star, but the lovely planet Venus.

As this realization breaks like a baptismal wave on your consciousness, you gradually begin to spiral downwards with the gentle motion of a dream into a beautiful starlit canyon which seems to lie directly below the white beams of Venus.

The canyon is deep and silent and dark, although you can see with shadowed clarity by the light of the moon and the stars. Here a Native American warrior awaits you, in traditional dress, bearing four shields.

Over his heart he wears a silver six-pointed star with an arrow-and-heart motif inscribed upon it. You know him to be a Warrior of Peace, charged to challenge and overcome those elements that arise within the sphere of human consciousness which seek to destroy the harmony and peace of the heart-centred soul.

He leads you to the midpoint of the canyon, where a great medicine wheel has been set out under the stars.

You walk with him to its centre, and he stands with you, tall and majestic, as you both look to the divine south.

He gives you one of his shields. It is red, inscribed with a wave formation and decorated with a crescent moon and wild turkey feathers. Three bands of orange wampum cross its face.

'The moon is the light which shines in the eternal summer of the south. Look through the dancing plant-forms and see Black Wolf Spirit. She will lead you to the source of wisdom.'

A garden, strange, wild and beautiful, seems to have grown up in the place of the south. You see a spectral black wolf, and allow your spirit to follow its lead deep into the garden-wilderness.

The garden is dancing, the plant forms lovely and ethereal around you. They sing with sweet chanting voices and emit strains of music. They clear suddenly under the crescent moon, and you come to a lagoon of pure water.

Under the moon, a mysterious figure repeatedly dives and re-emerges from the water, coming to rest on a crystal rock. You approach nearer and you see that she is a woman bearing the form of a mouse. Both shapes manifest in vivid coexistence. 'Who comes here to seek Diving Mouse Woman?' she asks.

Give her your name by saying it out loud.

You look into the eyes of Diving Mouse Woman, and see there the trust and innocence of a child; but you see also that these qualities cannot be exposed recklessly and thoughtlessly to the harshness of the outside world, but must be protected within the wisdom and the divine will of the spirit.

As you see this truth, you see also that you must be vigilant always to protect the child within you and all the children of the world, for from the eyes of Diving Mouse Woman there shines not only the sweetness of the infant but also the love and mighty care of Divine Mother. Diving Mouse Woman escorts you back to your past, and allows you to comfort and nurture the little child within your own nature.

Diving Mouse Woman begins to leap in and out of the water again; and this time you note her mouselike qualities, which surprise you with their scope and unexpectedness. You see that the mouse is endlessly resourceful, nimble and alert. Your human wits are not quick enough to follow its every movement. It is playful, curious, eager. It is meticulous and methodical. It is bold and daring, it pushes boundaries, it is cheeky. It has a celerity of movement and decision which is breathtaking, and a ferocity of will which can often outface human determination. It has an unquenchable zest for life; and yet its weakness is fear, which can make it panic blindly.

You see that Diving Mouse Woman is contained within the feeling body, the emotional body of your soul, and you see how this precious lagoon must be cherished and protected by the wise heart-light of your spirit, for it leaps with joyful life, and feeds your whole consciousness.

Black Wolf Spirit returns, and leads you back to the centre of the medicine wheel. Before you step over the threshold, your American Indian warrior guide says to you, 'Open your being to the lessons of this sacred orientation, and to all the beauty and the power and the revelations that come to your heart from the south.'

You obey his exhortation, and you see an enchanted city in the south, which is called Finias. Its sign is a spear, a fiery point which is destined to penetrate the heart so that it may wake and live, and slay all the dross of the being. It says: 'Remove the Veil of Fear!'

You step over the threshold and turn with your guide to the magical west.

He hands you the second shield, although you hold only one, as the first has blended with your soul and is no longer manifest. It is decorated with osprey feathers, and is inscribed with the symbol of a mountain with a single flowering tree growing from it. It is black with touches of gold, and crystals have been sewn into its deer-hide. It bears two black bands.

'Earthshine and the ancient signs of the zodiac light the fruitful autumn of the west,' says your guide. 'Look upon the Place of Stones, and follow Darting Bird Spirit to your destination.'

Darting Bird Spirit comes swooping into your field of vision, and you climb after her into the Place of Stones. Great boulders surround you, although they glimmer with half-hidden precious gems.

All around you the countryside bears the soft dun shades and fiery colours of autumn, and in the early morning sky a perfect, conical ring of pearly radiance sits like a crown upon heaven's dome. You know that it is the beautiful phenomenon of the Zodiacal Light.

Darting Bird Spirit leads you to a deep cave. You pass within. A great, shadowy bear is dancing in the mellow underworld dusk. You feel the dark, secret, potent and healing energies of the earth. You speak your name to the bear, saying it aloud.

The bear speaks: 'Dance with me, human soul, for I am your sister. I am Dreaming Bear.'

You dance with your sister bear, and as you dance you hear the beat of drums and the keening, exhilarating throb of Native American victory songs. Your dancing figures throw impossibly huge shadows on the great walls of the cave. The shadow of Dreaming Bear is no greater than your own.

As you dance, you sense that Dreaming Bear is indeed a great dreamer, for she spends almost half the year in hibernation, dreaming the Great Dream and studying the magical inner wisdom. You become aware of her power, of her massive stored energies. She is in truth a spirit of the sacred earth.

You think of the splitting of the atom and the untold power reserves held in the physical atoms of Mother Earth, you think of her wild stone heart, not cold and hard but loving, emanating warm and nurturing energy, like the ineffable beauty of her crystal self of which half her body consists. And yet the conundrum is that the weakness of the earth-state as humans experience it is inertia, powerlessness.

You think of your own physical body, your revered temple, the holy receptacle for divine spirit and its manifestation. You think of the sanctity of ancient things, and of how the ancient cycles must return, for nothing dies, but is only transformed as it passes through the body of the great Earth Mother. You feel how important it is to express Mother Earth's goodness, wholesomeness, her vitality and her beautiful energies by adhering to uncontaminated, natural foods, consumed without taint of cruelty, and of how these give good mental and emotional as well as physical health, keeping you firmly anchored in the rich and life-giving soil of the Eternal Now.

As Darting Bird Spirit returns and you take your leave of Dreaming Bear, you sense that the mysteries of the earth are far greater and deeper and more sublime than human imagination has ever conceived.

You find yourself back at the threshold again, ready to re-enter the heart of the medicine wheel.

Your guide says to you, 'Open your being to this magical orientation, and to all the beauty and the power and the revelations that have come to your heart from the west.'

You see the enchanted city of Murias twinkling in the mystery of the declining west; its sign is a miraculous hollow filled with water and fading light, the essence of earthshine which so mysteriously and dimly lights the heavens, the emanation of the veiled, inscrutable Earth Mother. It says: 'Remove the Veil of Shame!'

You step back into the middle of the medicine wheel, and your guide passes to you the third shield. Again, your hands are empty to receive it, because the south and the west shields have secreted themselves within your soul.

This shield is golden. It seems to flow with golden hair. It is decorated with golden eagle feathers. It is emblazoned with suns and with spirit forms in fountains of fire. It bears one yellow band upon which a single eye is engraved.

'Grandfather Sun lights the vernal skies of the Bright Land,' says your guide. 'Let Golden Warrior Woman lead the way, for your path penetrates the mysteries of the human heart.'

Beautiful, radiant, gracious and kindly, Golden Warrior Woman lifts you into the Bright Land on the currents of her sweet breath. She carries you to a mountaintop. There, wheeling above you in the blue, is a great golden eagle. 'Who is it that comes seeking Grandfather Eagle?' he cries.

You speak your name aloud and he drops to a rock in line with your brow centre, the very topmost peak of the mountain. He holds you in his vision with his sharp unblinking eye. 'You'll do,' he says, and launches suddenly into the air, giving three terrible shrieks.

They seem to resound in you and make you stagger back. When you regain your balance, the world has changed. You are in a sphere of inconceivably brilliant radiance. Your mind, your vision, your heart has never comprehended the possibility of such ecstasy, such glory, pulsing forth, giving forth, self-perpetuating, self-replenishing.

Beyond the disc, its source and its centre, is the perfect shape of a six-pointed star, calm as a vision of Paradise.

'You are in the heart of the sun,' says Grandfather Eagle. 'Dear one, do you not know that this is your own essence? How can you doubt yourself, your power to overcome, when this is your true home?'

You listen to Grandfather Eagle's words, and you feel a magnificent brotherhood, sisterhood, with every member of humanity and with all life. You see it go from you like a great ray of light, a beam of clarifying power. You see it cleansing away heavy sullied clouds into silver cascades of laughing endless light.

Grandfather Eagle bobs with joy. 'Those are clouds of misery and weariness which creep into the vision of the people on earth,' he says. 'Such clouds cannot resist the sun. The weakness of the east in human understanding is their way of perceiving death and decay. Humans do not see that it is but a transformation and a letting-go. They think it is a destination! The great sun laughs and dances at such folly! Now I will take you to the Place of Vision, so that you may be sure never to share in such blindness.'

A wheel of light rotates, and you are standing before a great pine tree. Beyond is a garden where the sun-spirits dance, of such wondrous pulchritude that you cannot see beyond the pine tree; you can only dimly know what is there in your deepest being.

The pine tree deposits a small, bright golden cone into your palm. Grandfather Eagle instructs you to press it to your brow centre.

'Now you are awakened,' he says. 'The gift from the sacred pine tree will enable you to see with the vision of your heart. Awaken the golden pine-cone by breathing quietly, by going to your heart-centre. Then your true eye will open, the all-seeing eye of your god-self, your gift from the Tree. Many call it the-mind-in-the-heart.'

Grandfather Eagle again rotates a wheel of light, you feel a rush of bright ether and you are back on the mountaintop.

There he teaches you how the eagle can look unflinchingly into the heart of the sun, how it soars above all lower things and overcomes their gravity-pull so that its nobility is never dishonoured, and how it takes the straight path into the grand heights, undistracted and undelayed, so that its vision is unconfined and all-embracing.

Grandfather Eagle teaches you that his kind are messengers from the Spirit, and that the Spirit is the heart of everlasting love.

Golden Warrior Woman comes to return you to your American Indian guide, gently wafting you on her fragrant currents of breath to the threshold of the eastern quarter of the Medicine Wheel.

Your guide addresses you: 'Open your being to the lessons of this mystical orientation, and to all the beauty and the power and the revelations that come to your heart from the east.'

You see the magical city of Gorias glittering in the rising sun, and a pure sword of flashing light which is its sign. You know that it is the sword of the spirit which must be wielded by every member of humanity, and that it points the way to humanity's future; and you hear it say, 'Remove the Veil of Self-Doubt!'

You step over the threshold and with your guide beside you, you turn at last to the sacred north. He gives you the last shield.

It is white, like a white sun. It is hung with white feathers, and decorated in wampum with birds and animals and stars. Four golden bands cross its face.

'The way of the north is lit by the mystery of the stars in its rapt Winter Dream. Star-Elk Spirit will show you the way,' says your guide.

A male elk appears before you, bearing magnificent antlers. You touch his nose hesitantly and he nuzzles your hand. Then he turns his great shoulders and walks into a shining mist.

You follow him, penetrating the shimmering mist, which dances around you in spears of rose, white, blue and green that glow with a deep glassy luminescence, like mirrored pools of light.

As you move further into these dancing, billowing lights, you begin to perceive many animal shapes. Some are well known to you, others are the great animals of the grassy plains of the world, and still others are completely unfamiliar, except that you recognize a fabulous or a mythical beast now and again.

You come to a ring of glimmering white rocks which seem suspended in the night sky. Nevertheless, there is a world here, and the landscape is covered in pure white snow.

The mists part and you see clearly that the ring of stones is peopled by tall and beautiful men and women, mighty of stature and dressed in ethereal flowing clothes similar in some respects to the ceremonial dress of the American Indians. Star-Elk Spirit speaks. 'These are the Star People. This sphere of the air is their Lodge. They will invoke White Buffalo Woman for you. You are honoured.'

The ceremony begins, flowing and pulsing in sweet and superb rhythm and song, moving in exhilarating cycles until a great white buffalo appears on the far horizon. It seems to descend from a group of stars softly glimmering with muted fire, a constellation you know to be the Pleiades, the Seven Sisters.

It half-rears on the skyline and then gallops towards you with a smooth, undulating motion.

As the buffalo draws closer you see that it is a woman who approaches you, a woman of miraculous beauty and grace, who bears within her form the presence of a great white buffalo. She is clothed in milk-white buffalo skins of fathomless purity and around her flows an aura of pearly essence and the white peace of newly fallen snow.

'Who is it that summons White Buffalo Woman?' she asks you, so that you speak aloud your name.

A deep stillness follows. In your spirit-body you kneel at the feet of White Buffalo Woman, for you see that here is Divine Mother, who, in her perfect love for her human child, gives of herself utterly and in entirety, for every part of the buffalo gave life to her children of the plains, gave them food, gave them clothes, gave them materials for constructing their tipis and bone-tools to facilitate their everyday lives.

Even the teeth of the buffalo gave them shamanic charms and protection. Behind the roving buffalo herds stood White Buffalo Woman, cherished spirit-mother to her people, endlessly bestowing her grace, her gifts, her essence.

Held within the tender white radiance of this great being, you realize deep within yourself that every human soul must learn to emulate her purity, her loving service, to give unstintingly of itself, holding nothing back, asking no return, lifting human giving above barter and control. And you see, also, that receiving White Buffalo Woman's gifts without appreciation and humility gives rise to an arrogant certainty, which is the weakness of the north for the human soul. You see that certainty must only be experienced and expressed concerning principles, never details.

Deeply you contemplate these things, deeply do you withdraw into the peace of your heart-centre to fathom the meaning, the beauty of these profound truths, for you see that meaning is beauty, and beauty is meaning. The presence of White Buffalo Woman touches your heart and makes you long to honour your own Beauty Path, the flight path of your spirit.

Star-Elk Spirit tosses his head and paws the ground, ready to escort you safely back to the centre of the medicine wheel.

White Buffalo Woman has taken her path to the stars and has returned to the bright Pleiades.

You give thanks to the graceful Star-People, recognizing that they are angels. As you follow Star-Elk Spirit back through the dancing, leaping, coloured mists, you realize that they are the Northern Lights and that you have penetrated their secret citadel.

You reach the threshold of the northern quarter of the medicine wheel. Your guide awaits. He says to you, 'Open your being to the lessons of this sacred orientation, and to all the beauty and the power and the revelations that come to your heart from the north.'

You see the fabled city of the spirit of the north played over by a deeply dreaming occult light, the visionary light of the Ancient of Days. It is Falias, and its sign is the stone of the transformation which is death, crowned by pale flickering fire. It says 'Banish the Veil

of Self-Will, for verily it is rooted in arrogance, narrowness and partial-sight! Flow with Divine Will, and
you shall spread peace and beauty across the world.'

You cross the threshold to your guide. He says to you,
'Now you must accept the Fifth Shield.'

Overhead, the peaceful stars and a new crescent moon
shine down into the silent, still, shadowed canyon. You
stand at the centre of the medicine wheel with your
guide.

As if a mist has fallen away from your eyes, you see
that you are standing in a glen of precious stones. Its
beauty and its peace are measureless.

'This is the Fifth City,' says your guide. 'It is the consecrated wedding-place of the soul and the spirit, where
they conjoin and become as one.

'Each gem is a solid structure of knowledge, of experience, that you have used to capture and contain the
light of your soul, the wisdom of the stars. These too
must pass away, so that only the living light remains —
dynamic, free, transformational.'

Looking up, you gaze at Venus shining in the night sky.
Your perception shifts and it is as if you are suddenly
looking up at a city of angels within the heart of the
bright planet.

As you watch, you perceive that the Glen of Precious
Stones magically becomes one with this angelic city,
as though there is an ascension and a descent and an
interpenetration.

You see that your guide is kneeling, and you kneel
beside him. Before you stands the figure of a man with
shining eyes, white-robed, bearing the sign of the
medicine wheel, the cross within the circle.

With great gentleness and love, he gives you your fifth shield. You see that it is made of light. It is decorated with the cross within the circle, the all-seeing eye, and a ring of hands. All its symbols are lit by stars, for this shield seems to contain the very galaxy itself.

'Make of your soul a song to the Great Spirit,' the white-robed man says. 'Pray to the winds; the Great Spirit will hear you. Pray to the galaxy, set your light-body walking on the Milky Way; the Great Spirit will bless you. Let the sun and the moon guide you, and let your spirit dwell often upon the beauty and mystery of Venus, for she has much to teach the stumbling children of earth. But above all things, turn again and again to the star in your heart, for that is the Great Spirit's source. Do these things, and you shall know peace.'

He blesses both you and your guide; as the fifth city recedes again into mystery you stand at the centre of the simple medicine wheel.

'We have met with Heah-Wah-Sah, the Healer, Lord of Wind and Water, the holy Prophet-God of the American Indian tribes,' says your guide. 'We have met with He-Who-Will-Come-Again.'

As day breaks in the cool pure air of the canyon and Venus shines silver below the brilliant circle of the early morning sun, a deep knowledge is conveyed to you that humanity itself is standing on the brink of a new dawn which will bring deep and abiding peace to all the nations and to the round rim of the world, from north to south, from east to west.

Feel the vision comforting, healing and inspiring every level of your being, so that you take up your life anew as a warrior of peace, guided always by the wise and peace-making warrior eternally by your side.

Gently return to normal waking consciousness, seal your centres (crown, brow, throat, heart, solar plexus) with the bright silver cross in a circle of light, and earth yourself if necessary.

Affirm:

I walk my beauty path in peace.

Peace flows to me from the stars.

I am a warrior of peace.

CHAPTER THREE

THE SEVEN SECRET HEALING IMPLEMENTS OF THE SOUL

These seven instruments are secret because they are secreted within us. They are:

- the rose
- the star
- the rainbow chalice
- the rainbow bridge
- the nous
- the sword
- the chakras of the hands

The Angel Samandiriel

We must find each secret implement within our heart-aware-ness – the point of intelligence within the heart. Before we can do this, we need to call on the faculty of our imagination. The great angel who blesses, fecundates, and lights the stars of the imagination is the mighty Samandiriel.

As we explore each of the sacred implements of the soul, we will call often on Samandiriel to assist us in our creative visualization. It would serve you well to use these opportunities to build your own personal relationship with Samandiriel and to change an acquaintanceship into a friendship. Of course, in our dealings with angels, we must always remember that a degree of the impersonal is necessary in our relationship with them. This does not mean that we must have no personal feelings for our angel friends, and that they have no personal feelings for us. It just means that we must never cramp our friendships with angels into the constrictions and limitations of our ego, always bearing in mind that both angel and human work together for the benefit of all, and that in our associations with the angels we must impose no horizon on our vision which blocks our consciousness of the greater good, the bigger picture. So, for the sake of your development as an angel healer, get to know Samandiriel as we work through the following exercises and make of this benevolent and richly gifted shining one a loving friend and ally.

The Rose

We find the rose in our heart chakra. It sends forth a fragrance that can heal all beings, that can heal the world. It is our very heart of hearts, the uttermost centre of our being. We will find that it is connected with the 'nous' (*see* below) and with the divine figure 5, the sacred number of our planet.

Roses are built on a calyx of five sepals. If you sketch a figure around the sepals, joining their tips, a pentagram appears, the sacred pentagram upon which the structure of the human form is created, with its four limbs and head. If we stand with legs apart and arms outstretched, we make evident our pentagrammatical form, in which every single line declares what is known as the Golden Mean, or Divine Proportion: the infusion of the balance, peace and perfect justice of the essence of the Godhead. From ancient times, the rose has often been depicted at the heart of a cross. This signifies that from the garnerings of lives lived upon the sacrificial cross of time and matter, there blooms in every human soul divine consciousness – the true spiritual essence of the rose.

A profound mystery dwells in the image of the rose that blooms at the very heart of the cross: it is matter's innermost secret. The rose is a symbol of the heart and of human and divine love. When it blooms upon the cross of matter in an individual's life, the spiritual essence pervades the earthly being. In esoteric understanding, such a man or woman is seen to be 'Christed', or expressing the divine life. The rose is an emblem of matter, and life lived through matter, brought to perfection. When this point is reached, matter is no longer just an emanation of spirit, imperfect because it exists such a long way off from the divine centre; it becomes spirit itself. It has returned to the centre, to the heart, it is once again heart. It has come home and is no longer perishable and corruptible. That is matter's secret, and is the measure of our task here on earth as spiritual beings clothing ourselves in matter in order to extend the frontiers, create new dimensions of perfected creation.

The rose is fathomless in its beauty, its meaning and its promise. The use of the rose as a meditation symbol plays a vital part in our reclamation of our divine essence, our becoming fully human. When resentment, anger, apathy or unresponsiveness arising from any source clouds our ability to meditate, the rose will unlock our resistance.

Rose Healing

Imagine a dew-touched rose, pink as the first flush of sunrise, as though placed by a divine hand in your heart-centre… the shining hand of the Angel Samandiriel. Breathe in its healing fragrance, and delight in the rose temple that Samandiriel builds around you… No matter what the outer conditions of life, this gentle focus on the rose in the heart will bring peace, a fount of purity and wellbeing and the realization that we are eternally linked to the source of Love. It will bring to you a realization of its essence beyond the stumblings and limitations of mere words and thoughts. It will lead you to that point of peace 'which passeth all understanding'.

When you have become truly aware of the rose in your heart, you will realize that it is much, much more than just a beautiful healing and meditation symbol. It is a power in your life, part of the potency of your being. You can literally breathe forth its fragrance at the subtle spiritual level to bring healing, calm, and a pure breath of magic to any situation in which you find yourself; but it must be borne in mind that the essence of the rose is the essence of giving. Giving forth the sunlight of our being from the heart ignites the power of the rose. Then we walk in a world of repose, beauty and meaning, and put on our true selfhood, our true humanity.

This true self is depicted at the heart of every rose by its circle of golden stamens. It is a sigil, written in matter itself, of the 'mind in the heart', the intuitive mind which is linked to the 'pure reason' of divine love, found in the heart-centre.

There is a power and an essence distilled by the rose that is beyond all earthly understanding. It is there for us to draw upon, to enter into and to receive as a gift from heaven.

The Star

The spiritual star within our heart is the most vital part of ourselves. Tuning in to the star summons the divine light in our being. We are protected, we can give forth healing and blessing, and our consciousness is transformed.

To attune to the star, go to the heart-centre (just touching it lightly can help our mind to rest there) and begin to focus gently on the breath. Imagine that you are drawing in to your being the golden-white light of Goddess-God, and exhaling all the anxiety and distractions of the earthly life. After a little while you will find that you are both inhaling and exhaling this perfect spiritual light.

Star Meditation

Imagine a six-pointed star shining in your heart. It is composed of two equilateral triangles, one pointing upwards and one pointing downwards. The two triangles merge and the star blazes forth, without any inner divisions.

See yourself standing in the heart of the star, and see the star shining from your own heart. It also shines above your head, down onto your crown. These three realities all occur simultaneously, so that you become one with the star.

The spiritual star is connected to the Pole Star, to the Star of Bethlehem, and to the Sphere of John – an exalted realm wherein the Holy City (the glorious, angel-lit civilization which is waiting to descend to earth and supplant our current age of darkness and suffering as soon as we allow it to do so) is contained.

The star is our point of entry to the Holy City. It is the point of our being where magic resides: the full glory of the spirit. It is used in conjunction with the breath to breathe in and breathe out blessing, healing, protection, divine inspiration. The thought, the breath, the loving intention within directs the light to its chosen destination. It is the power of Goddess-God, it is the power of the divine Son-Daughter, it is the power of pure love. Used correctly, without selfishness, the star is indeed all-powerful. It is a symbol of the human being made perfect – the fully human being.

The teacher White Eagle says of the star:

> Where the star shines by the will and through the
> love of earthly men and women, the effect over
> chaos and disorder, war, and all the evils in the
> world can be truly magical.

From *The Book of Starlight*, White Eagle

Take every opportunity to use the star! We bypass our divine
heritage if we ignore it and receive its light only unconsciously.
The star burns with pure spiritual fire, and it cannot be put to
evil or selfish use. We can use it to beautify and inspire our lives,
to protect and heal ourselves, and to bring joy and vision to our
daily tasks. But, most of all, we can use it to give those gifts of the
spirit to others, to all humanity, to the planet herself. And when
there are sufficient numbers of us who will daily ignite that
mystical light, despite the blunderings of politicians and the
spectres of hatred and carnage, the world will change beyond all
recognition.

If you experience any difficulty in visualizing the star,
remember to call on Samandiriel. Let this shining angel become
a spiritual mirror. See your heart-centre reflected in its depths,
with the star shining there. Samandiriel will help to create it.

The Rainbow Chalice

The rainbow chalice is the heart. Call on Samandiriel to fire
your vision, and use the breath and the magical symbol of the
six-pointed star to find it. See this beautiful chalice of light in
the centre of the heart chakra, where the mystical rose dwells.
The rose becomes the holy fragrance, the holy breath within the
chalice, which gives it its form and its healing magic. The star
gives it the potency of the spirit.

When we need to send out healing, or when we need to heal ourselves by silently bathing in the light of the heart, we can draw near to the angels and ask them to reflect the heavenly colours of the rays of creation within the white-golden star of the heart.

Let the star rise from your heart to above your head, revealing the pearly chalice. It is overflowing with light. Call on the angels to shine a colour or colours into the fountain of light spilling from the chalice. Ask them out loud and outright.

These colours might be:

Rose – the colour of heavenly love and reassurance;

Angelic golden-yellow – the colour of happiness, which dispels negativity and eases harsh mindsets;

Soft apple green – the colour of deep sympathy and understanding;

Summer sky-blue – the colour of peace and relief from pain;

Sunset red-orange – which gives vitality and stimulation;

Amethyst – which gives endurance, inner strength, and freedom from the enslavement of addictions;

Indigo – which enhances spiritual devotion and soothes relationships;

Pearl – which brings the balm of motherly love;

Gold – which brings the protection of fatherly love;

Magenta – which stabilizes and steadies, comforts and balances.

Let each colour wash over you in a flood, encircling you gently in a clockwise direction. Never see the colours as brash and opaque, but rather as pure, radiant and delicate, like jewel colours, flashing with a subtle vividness.

It is unwise to bathe the whole aura in deep, strong, earthy colours. When you commence your healing work, put the colour emanation into the hands of the angels; they will know the brightness or the softness of the hue you require.

The Rainbow Bridge

This mystic bridge is the bridge between the spirit and the soul. It is where the 'nous' is located (*see* below) and its point of entry is within the heart chakra.

The soul is the very first body in which spirit clothes itself in order to make a stairway down to the realms of matter, the physical body being the outermost body. The little individualized spark of the Divine Spirit is clothed in the soul, but it also has to build the greater soul through its experiences in matter. It comes down into incarnation wearing the soul body, but the spirit and the soul together have to set to work to build the great Soul Temple in the higher worlds. Over many, many lives this structure is gradually constructed and perfected, until it becomes worthy to house the spirit, now expanded to a great light through self-awareness, which eventually becomes God-consciousness.

When the temple is ready, the soul becomes utterly translucent and the spirit shines through her and is consummate with her, the sacred marriage takes place and the soul and the spirit become as one. But for the soul and the spirit to be unobstructed in their communion, the antahkarana – the beautiful rainbow bridge, has to be realized. Then it can connect our little everyday self with the glorious light, seven-rayed, of the Divine. It is then that the personality no longer stands in the way of our becoming a radiant being, a being who emits light, instead of imprisoning us in selfhood (or isolation) with issues of its own.

The potency of prayer, of invocation of the highest consciousness of which we can conceive, is hugely important to the process of building the rainbow bridge, because the great rule of creation is that its mode of being is reciprocal. The lesser and the greater, the lower and the higher, the younger and the elder brethren must consciously work together, the lesser and the lower ever invoking, by its own conscious free will, the grace and blessing, the infusion of the higher and greater.

This is the fundamental way in which creation works, its elementary design (of course, 'fundamental' and 'elementary' are words which are only appropriate for us to use at our particular earthly stage of development; they cannot really apply to a design so stupendous as the cosmos). It embodies the principle that energy always flows from the stronger source to the weaker source. It is the principle of endless, unstinting giving upon which creation rests. It is Christ saying, 'Sell all you have, and give to the poor,' meaning the poor in spirit. This scientific fact, energy flowing from the stronger to the weaker source, is a reflection of the great cosmic law which is worked out in the act of prayer or invocation.

So prayers and the act of prayer, the act of invocation, contain this great cosmic secret: that they work with Divine Spirit, via the angels and other higher beings, to construct the exquisitely beautiful antahkarana, the rainbow bridge of the soul. This is why, of course, the promised pot of gold is found where the rainbow meets the earth. This is the solar gold from the spirit that the soul brings back to the little earthly personality, the solar gold that must indeed be rooted in the earth, in matter itself, by the soul, and breathed upon and fostered by her, until the earthly personality grows into a being of gold, a gold which is surrendered up, in its turn, to release greater light, more of the light of Goddess-God, in the little individualized spark of the human spirit. And so the rainbow bridge faithfully fulfills the potential of its bilateral nature.

Locating the Rainbow Bridge

To find the rainbow bridge, gently rest your awareness in your heart, and see the star blazing there in white light.

Call the Angel Samandiriel to your side, so that you might construct the bridge together, and, when it is built, traverse its wonder, hand in hand.

Breathe three cycles of the Mother's Breath (*see* Chapter Two), and begin to see a line of white light ascending from your heart to your throat chakra, which spins and glows now with a globe of light, shining white and throwing out brilliant whirling glints of a sweet, vivid lilac colour.

Now see the line of white light extend to your brow chakra, where the globe of white light again begins to spin, throwing off rose-hued sparks of brilliance.

Continue your cycles of breathing, and see the line of white light rising to your first brow chakra, at the top of your forehead in the middle. This also begins to spin, becoming a globe of pure white light.

Now see the brilliant white light form a line across your scalp to the centre, where your second crown chakra is located in the middle of the brain. As this chakra begins to spin, it also becomes a sphere of bright white light.

Become aware that the line of light from your heart to your throat, from your throat to your brow, from your brow to the top of your forehead, from there to your crown, is forming a great bridge of light.

The first end starts in the heart and runs through the higher chakras until it reaches the point in the middle of the brain. From there it extends into eternity, into infinite expansion, forming the arch of the traditional rainbow.

As you watch and realize its presence, the two crown chakras begin to rain an exquisite light-show of rainbow colours onto the bridge, and the bridge itself is transformed into a bow of brilliant crystalline rainbow colours, seven-hued and yet many times more than seven-hued.

This is the rainbow bridge, the antahkarana stretching between the soul and the spirit. It is yours to summon whenever you will, in the knowledge that the rainbow is truly a circle, and within that circle your spirit and your soul will find true union, and rejoice together in the wedding ring.

The Nous

The 'nous' is the mind in the heart, that centre of intelligence which includes intuition and sensibility within its compass. It is the subject of a profoundly significant teaching given in The Gospel of Mary Magdalene, an enigmatic and beautiful little text which was discovered in a Cairo antiquities shop by a German academic in the closing years of the 19th century. Half of the manuscript had been torn away, so that only ten pages were still extant.

However, under the guidance of Mary Magdalene, Margaret Bailey and I were enabled to tell her full story and to reveal the entire Magdalene gospel text in our recent book, *The Secret Teachings of Mary Magdalene*. This made all clear, and revealed what the 'nous' truly is. In the Mary gospel, Jesus speaks of it as the point between the soul and the spirit. It connects our head and our heart-centres via the antahkaranah, the rainbow bridge which links heaven and earth, but it is centred in the heart. If we remember that the soul is the first, pristine body of the indwelling spirit (it has to be kept pristine) – the spirit that is the 'little spark' which has come down to earth to learn to grow into a fully fledged spiritual being (an apt description, because we do develop wings) – we can understand that they are virtually one. But they are not quite one until the mystical marriage has taken place, which can only happen after soul ascension has been accomplished.

The spark of spirit, our true self, is wrapped in many bodies, many dense layers or skins, and we have to penetrate each one before we can find it and release it. The question arises as to who is the 'I' that strives to find the spirit, if the spirit is our true self. The answer, in simplistic form, is that the 'I' which is our consciousness is a mirror image of the little spark, fed down to the everyday level of awareness through a strand of the soul, the mirror image which must reverse if it is to become 'fully human' (a repeated expression which occurs throughout the gospel text). The 'little spark' constantly calls the mirror image back home. We find our way home to our spirit through our soul. This is why it is so vital to nurture our soul, according it high honour and ministering to it so that we might find our way to the Source, the spirit.

Therefore the 'nous' does lie in the soul ('The eye of the vision is in the soul', lines 2–3, p.1, The Gospel of Mary Magdalene), but it is also the connecting point between the soul and the spirit, the magical threshold and doorway. That is why Jesus tells us, 'Where the nous is, there lies the treasure.' (line 15, p.10, The Gospel of Mary Magdalene). Nevertheless, we ourselves have to make the connection; we have to marry the soul and the spirit via our own aspiration and free will. It is a procedure we must initiate – it is not done for us. When at last the soul opens the magical doorway and fully admits the light of the spirit, then we become 'fully human'. We become a God-man or God-woman, the perfect being Goddess-God envisaged when we were first created or breathed forth from the Godhead, rather than the reverse or mirror image, the 'beast-man' or 'beast-woman' which we are until our soul ascends to meet and marry our spirit. Therefore, the soul (Beauty) leads forth the 'beast' (our unrealized self) through the magic door or mirror (the 'nous') so that it becomes the glorious God-being, and we are baptized by light into our 'fully human' state.

This magical doorway (the 'nous') between the soul and the spirit is the mind-in-the-heart, the point of peace within. Most importantly, we discover its location through our breath. Our breath is indeed magical and deeply sacred 'celestial fire'. Our breath is the key.

This 'vision within the soul' which is the 'nous', or the heart-mind, can not only see and be seen (it sees the vision and the vision is seen), it can hear and be heard. First, we start to listen to it by listening to and gently focusing on our own breath. The gentle rhythmic sound of our breathing, if listened to in reverence as in an act of prayer, will take us into the Silence, becoming 'the breath of Silence' (line 8, p.1, The Gospel of Mary Magdalene). Once this has happened, we will be able to hear in the highest and truest sense. Our inner faculties will spring into life. We were born as if deaf and blind to the beautiful spiritual realities of our existence. The mystical grace of the 'nous' restores what was lost to us, and releases us from our grim prison.

We see that the heart chakra holds the wonders of the star, the rose, the rainbow chalice, and the 'nous'. All are aspects of the one glory – our living spirit, the gift of God that is God within us. Yet the 'nous' is the key. We might call it the breath of the star, the breath of the rose; for it is the magic, the spirit, the radiance of the star and the fragrance of its heart of hearts, the rose, that sounds the creative Word that opens the door for the soul onto the spiritual worlds. It is this magic, this fragrance, that marks the exact site of the 'nous'. We have to be able to go within and reach this point, to home into it like a returning bird. 'Where the nous is, there lies the treasure.' Wings of peace will carry you there.

Ask the bright Angel Samandiriel to help you find this greatest of all treasures, the point of peace and wonder within that is the 'nous', the Silmarillion of the soul.

The Sword

Within the true sword of the spirit lies the Word (s-word). John's gospel opens with the statement 'In the beginning was the Word; and the Word was with God, and the Word was God.' This unconscionable power of the Word is the power of the sword.

The sword flashes within us. We might say it is the power of the spine, of that ramrod of light that connects us to heaven and earth so that, as spirit earthed in flesh, it is possible for us to be, to survive, as the entities we are. We must align and ally our own sword with that of Archangel Michael if we want it to be safe, sure and sound. We do this simply by making the request in prayer to him each time before we begin work with the sword. Additionally, ask Michael to bless your sword and your healing endeavours. Ask him to place his hand over yours as you use the sword.

In our healing work, we wield the sword with tender caution. It flashes brilliant blue-silver. We hold it boldly and firmly in our right hand, and with its brilliantly gleaming silver blade we gently cut away from our patient, whether they are present or absent, any unhealthy condition of the mind or soul that might have taken a stranglehold there. Obsession, addiction, inner slaveries and unsavouriness, all eventually loosen their hold and fall away on the application of the blessed s-word of the spirit.

One important factor to bear in mind when we are giving angel healing is that people can sometimes become very attached to their illnesses! Patients can grow quite fond of them, and discuss them constantly, forever gathering new information about them and focusing on little else. When this is the case, the patient needs gentle counselling in the art of letting go of their illness. It is all too easy for sickness to become a perverse source of comfort and status, giving sufferers identity and importance, and a course by which to run their lives. The sword of Michael is very much required in such cases, and our role as educators has to be brought to the fore. Avoid harshness or tactlessness, of course, but do explain that it is only when we are truly sick of our sickness that we can let it go, and allow the angels to usher in the required healing forces!

Occasionally, we will encounter those who really do not wish to let go of their malady under any circumstances. We cannot impose our will 'for their own good' and attempt to bombard them out of their negative thinking, however much we may be tempted to do so! As healers working with the angels, we must always have a thoroughly conscientious respect for our patients' free will. It is imperative never to force an issue. Continue to give comfort and seek to alleviate their pain, but it is unwise to expend a great deal of time and energy on such cases, not only for your own sake, but also because in doing so we tend to feed the root of their problem.

Unfortunately, such patients often make a point of demanding huge tracts of time and energy! Be firm, and call on the angels to help you discriminate and use your time and energy wisely. Sophia is the great angel of wisdom, and she will come to your aid in this task as in many others. Wise conservation of our energy is one of the first lessons we must learn as angel healers, otherwise a situation will develop similar to all others that develop around bad economy!

Never wield this healing and cleansing sword in anger or for selfish purposes, because it will turn against you. Whenever you hold the sword of Michael, the healing angels and the Divine Spirit which animates them enter with you into a pact of trust. They trust your honour, your resolution, and your discretion. To betray this pact is a gross dereliction of duty, so we always let the highest and purest knight within step forward in our soul whenever we make use of the s-word. This great Warrior of

Peace, with whom we became acquainted in the Starlit Canyon meditation (*see* Chapter Two), will keep you from stumbling.

The Chakras of the Hands

Not every patient will welcome the laying on of hands. Nevertheless, whether or not we use them physically, the hands are among our greatest healing tools. They can convey forces, colours, angelic ministration, even without coming into contact with those who suffer.

It is important to remember always that the angels fashioned our hands in their own image. This is not just the expression of a sentiment or an appealing image, but the exact truth. We must learn to revere our hands as agents of healing through which the angels can manifest.

When actively engaged in angel healing, we must ensure that the exercises given in Chapter One (*see* Healing Hands, page 11) are adhered to carefully. Wash your hands before and after each angel healing session, both physically and spiritually, using the little ceremony of The Angel of the Chaste Hands or Starlight Hand-Bathing. Combine the two ceremonies, or perform them one after the other, to ensure a beautiful revivification and purification of your hands' energies. Practise the second part of the Vivaxis ceremony (*see* Locating the Vivaxis, page 14) once each day, so that the chakras in your hands and feet are cleansed, invigorated and balanced by the circuits of light described.

Finally, when you are ready to begin your healing services, call on Archangel Raphael, his circle of healing angels, and the Angels of Mercy to bless your hands, and imbue them with healing energy. Michael, Gabriel and Zadkiel are the Angels of Mercy, and you can supplicate them by name as well as by their title.

Whilst this book was underway, a friend who is an angel healer and a conduit for their messages to humanity, sent me the details of a very remarkable and beautiful healing ceremony given to her by the Archangel Zadkiel, who has charge of the Violet Flame (*see* Chapter One) and who is one of the three great Angels of Mercy. It is so rewarding and replenishing that I would like to offer it here, as a gift from Dianne Pegler for the benefit of all those who work with the angels to help others, and who sometimes find that their own energies are depleted and need restoring. Of course, patients will greatly benefit from it too.

Archangel Zadkiel's Message and Healing Ceremony for Light Workers

'I AM Zadkiel.

'I AM The Archangel of the Gold, Silver and Violet Flame and my energies will transmute all negativity in your life, Spiritual, Physical and Emotional, if you allow me. I will transform your life to one of sublime joy and vibrational harmony with your Creator.

'I AM come in answer to the Clarion Call to The Violet Flame from many of those incarnate on Planet Earth at this time.

'I AM come to offer healing, recuperation and respite from the many pressures which are seeming to over-whelm and overburden many Light Workers. So much so, that while The Ascension (2012/13) is never in doubt, there are many who are not enjoying the esca-lation path as they should for one reason or for many reasons.

'The Violet Flame will address the imbalance and The Angelic Hierarchy have sent this message to Planet Earth. You will no doubt notice many references to invoking The Violet Flame or references to St Germain of The Violet Flame at this time and this is, of course, no coincidence.

'You have heard of the spiritual adage, *As Above So Below*, so many times, perhaps now more than ever.

'It is time now to *really* embrace this philosophy into the very soul of you, Dear Ones. The Violet Flame will help you to do so and with speed. We have heard your impassioned pleas and are responding.

'In particular, we are reaching out to Light Workers who have been on The Spiritual Path for many years now. You are the ones who appear even more burdened than those who know nothing of this very special and enlightened path. There is a feeling of 'losing your way', of knowing so much and knowing nothing at all. The more you learn, the more complicated your path appears to be. I say to you, become as little children once again, and you will release the tensions and pressures that beset you.

'I AM come to offer you solace in a meaningful way, Dear Ones. We begin...

'I call upon Archangel Michael to offer you protection and purification. Invoke this mighty Archangel to absorb all negative cords and attachments clinging to your aura and etheric body. Visualize Archangel Michael scanning your mind, body and spirit and removing all those unwanted memories, hurts, seeming failures, rejections, guilty and shameful thoughts from you. See his flaming sword cleansing your aura and etheric body and sealing it with blazing blue Light as if covering you with His own cobalt-blue cloak of protection. Feel the absolute peaceful bliss of this cleansing and ask Archangel Michael to seal your aura and etheric body permanently.

'I AM Zadkiel and I invoke the other Archangels to now draw near and to bow before you in greeting.

'Our beautiful rays have formed a rainbow bridge and we invite you to cross over this rainbow bridge into an exquisite Healing Sanctuary which has been created in the Angelic Realm to grant you peace, Dear Ones. We invite you to call upon The Violet Flame and to cross over the rainbow bridge very often in the coming weeks and months. By doing so, you will strengthen your spiritual purpose as never before and with joy, love, peace and the perfect vibrational balance of The Creator and The Angelic Realm.

'You are returning to Atlantis, Dear Ones, for in truth you were there when it was the wondrous city of healing and knowledge. The Atlantis you are now returning to is one formed in The Angelic Realm and will never succumb to negative energies as it did before. One of the reasons that many Light Workers are falling prey to negativity, to addictions, to illness, to overwork and fatigue is that the remembrances of their past life in early Atlantis remains deep within their very Being. They remember so well the sublimeness of their life in Atlantis and the horror of when everything changed.

'I AM Zadkiel and I say to you The Violet Flame can and will transmute this memory and release it once and for all from your consciousness.

'You are now crossing over the rainbow bridge and you are now walking towards the Great White Marble Healing Dome. You are dressed as you did when you walked the streets of the early Atlantis for you offici-ated in the Great White Healing Dome. You are wearing a simple gold crown with a crystal droplet hanging over your Third Eye. You are wearing a simple gown and cloak trimmed with gold braid.

'The feeling of "coming home" is catching at your eyes and throat as you remember it all so well.

'You enter the magnificence of the Great White Healing Dome. It is, of course, completely round with the white marble walls towering upwards culminating in a spectacular, circular cut glass window at the apex. It seems as though that window is even above the clouds in the sky!'

Directly below the circular ceiling window, on the floor, is a huge quartz crystal lovingly worked into one million facets to catch the Light from The Creator. This crystal sits on a plinth filled with Sacred Healing Waters and slowly turns to catch The Light, showering the Great White Healing Dome with millions of bursts of colours all around the walls and floor. The walls of the Great White Healing Dome rotate in the opposite direction to the crystal. The effect of complete and utter disorientation is liberating, breathtaking, and uplifts You to become as One with your Creator.

Your gold crown is removed. A beautiful circlet of amethyst, rose quartz, emerald, ruby, lapiz lazuli and clear white quartz crystal is placed upon your head and your cloak is removed.

There are Angels in this Angelic Atlantis who guide you to a marble healing bed. You feel yourself gently lifted and placed on this bed. You brace yourself to slightly resist the hard and cool surface. You realize, however, that you are suspended within the marble bed on a taut cotton hammock which effortlessly supports the weight of your body, leaving your head to gently flop.

The hammock is joined to the marble bed by strings

and strands which have been carefully formed to resonate perfectly with every single particle of you even down to the last eyelash! There is a string or strand to resonate with your organs, your skin, your hair, your vertebrae and bones, your eyes and ears, your muscles, your blood, every cell and all your senses.

The pure air of the Great White Healing Dome supports your head so that it may be healed independently from your body. Your soul, of course, is nurtured by the entire experience.

'I AM Zadkiel of The Violet Flame and I say, "Let The Healing Begin." '

As you lie there, suspended on the Marble Healing Bed, the million-faceted quartz crystal begins to rotate a little faster, causing billions of bursts of Light to whirl and dance rapidly around the walls and floor of the Great White Healing Dome. The strings and strands of the Marble Bed you lie suspended upon begin to hum, entoning deep vibration as they are energized by the speed of The Light. There is a feeling of complete weightlessness such as you never dreamt possible. It is a transcendence of Mind, Body and Soul experience. The healing is complete. You are vibrating in tune with Your Creator. Your song is the song of all Creation.

You lie there in a state of bliss and absolute healing.

Lie there for as long as you want. You feel that you *never*, *ever* want this to finish.

You hear Archangel Zadkiel intone: 'I AM The Gold, Silver and Violet Flame,' over and over as you lie in your bliss.

'I AM Zadkiel.

'You have called and I have answered.

'I Am The Violet Flame and this healing ritual will be made known to many.

'It will empower all those who call upon the trans-forming energies of The Violet Flame.

'I AM Zadkiel.'

Channelled by Dianne Pegler,
3 a.m. GMT, 16 May 2007

CHAPTER FOUR

RAPHAEL & HIS COMPANY OF HEALING ANGELS

As dedicated angel healers, we must make the acquaintance of the great angel Raphael and his circle of healing angels. A loving and creative relationship with this great company is essential to our work. The Archangel Raphael wields the caduceus, a mighty staff composed of two opposite serpents coiling and twisting round one another until their heads meet under the top of the staff, which comprises the extended wings of a swan, associated with the right and the left ventricles of the brain. These denote the two different aspects of consciousness, the sacred feminine and the sacred masculine, which dwell within us and which we, as human beings (together with all things) embody. The harmonizing of these opposites into a single stream of perfected consciousness is the whole task of our life on earth. All healing flows from this concept, and the angel Raphael is the shepherd and the facilitator of the healing process. This great angel has worked with all who walked the earth on healing missions, and especially with the divine Christ couple, Jesus and Mary Magdalene.

Our Angelic Name

Before we begin to draw close to Raphael in thought and meditation, it is important to establish our own angelic name. This is distinct from the name of our guardian angel and the name of the group of angels who have us under their care, which we can discover via various methods (*see* my book, *Your Guardian Angel*, for the appropriate exercises). What we are searching for here differs in that we need to discover the particular sound or name within us that resonates with our own angel essence, and with which the angels can immediately link when we call on them in our healing work or in our daily lives.

We might think that the human entity stands far below the angels in the ranks of spiritual evolution. In our present state this may be so, but the angels themselves reassure us that 'the spiritual immortal ego [of humanity] shines forth with a splendour and a power equalled only amongst the highest of the angel ranks.' This is wonderful news, humbling knowledge indeed, because the glory of 'the highest of the angel ranks' is beyond our earthly conception.

The name we seek will, with its resonances, remind us at the profoundest level of our being of our true heritage, and will call on the angelic quality that dwells in the deeps of that many-splendoured 'spiritual immortal ego' to rise and blaze forth, and shine its light into our imprisoned earthly self so that our angel work takes place 'out of the box' or the prison which normally confines us, until we at last learn to overstep its barriers.

Finding our Angelic Name

It is wise to ground yourself for this exercise. This can be done by sitting with both feet on the floor and imagining strong, vigorous roots growing from the centre of both feet (the feet chakras) deep down into the heart of the earth, where she receives them with love and allows their prehensile grip to fix into her.

Light a white candle (in imagination if this is more convenient) and dedicate it to the great angel Gethel (Geth-elle) who has charge over hidden things.

Create the form of the star in your heart and withdraw to the centre of this peaceful radiance.

Begin to softly chant the name Gethel.

Harmonize the sound with your breathing until a feeling of spiritual calm gently releases you from everyday consciousness.

Say aloud: 'Angel Gethel, beloved one of the Supreme Light, reveal to me my hidden name, the one that vibrates with my angel essence and resonates with the angelic realms.'

In your serene and purified state, listen closely (but take care not to try too hard or to tensely strain after what is given to you) until you perceive a name.

As soon as you are confident that you have heard clearly, withdraw from meditation, seal your centres, and as you blow out your candle, thank Gethel, the Angel who has charge over hidden things.

Don't worry if your newly discovered name sounds rather extraordinary! The angelic language encompasses many more dimensions than our babel of earth languages, and you may receive a peculiar sound rather than what you might think of as a name in conventional terms! Sometimes, a person is given the name of an actual angel. If this is the case, it is always worth consulting an angel dictionary to look up your angelic name, as the qualities of the specified angel may give you an insight into the latent virtues which wait to be developed within you, and that call you to unfold their shining potential with the sweet unearthly voice of the angels.

Archangel Michael's Purifying Fire

Before we begin our mission of angel healing, there is a short and simple ceremony we need to undergo. The ceremony takes the form of an initiation, and although it sounds alarming, it is actually quite safe! It involves calling forth the holy fire of Michael, from our feet upwards, until we are cleansed of all our accumulated dross. This dross consists of impure psychic matter which has gathered in our aura and chakras over many lifetimes, and which, to some degree, repeatedly appears in these locations each time we reincarnate until we consciously oust it. This psychic matter is created by pandering to what is unwise and gross in our nature. We can free ourselves of the impurity created by our past self-indulgences by working through the following ceremony.

The Dance of the Two Dragons (1)

To perform this ceremony we need to call on our spiritual will. We should not be afraid of the power of our will. We shall be calling on that will to manifest itself which is attuned to the highest of the high, to Divine Spirit, not our own self-will, which, as it has no vision and is not sourced in love, inevitably trips us up! We can also address the same ceremony to Brigid so that the male and female principles informing our willpower remain in balance.

> Create the star in the heart with your imagination. Let it grow until it contains you in its heart. Stand within the protection of the star throughout this ceremony.

> Say: 'Archangel Michael, Angelic Lord of Fire, be with me and protect me during this ritual. Please bless and oversee my endeavour.'

> Hold forth your right hand, and see an unlit torch there in your grasp.

Say: 'Archangel Michael, light my torch with heavenly fire!'

See the torch blazing with spiritual fire. Its glory out-shines the sun.

Say: 'This ignited torch is my higher will. With it I invoke the spiritual fire to take light at my feet, and engulf each of my subtle bodies in purifying, renewing flame.'

Lower the torch to your feet, letting it rest there. See a glowing fire spring to life beneath your feet. See its tongues of flame rise in a great column around you.

Stand in its brilliant centre, letting them sweep through you, hearing the roaring song of the flames as they take into themselves all the contaminated energy which has burdened you for so long. Rejoice in this cleansing, knowing that your heart embraces it, and it is what your spirit longs for.

As the flames dance around you, know that you are truly a dragon, a creature of spiritual fire. Like King Arthur, you are the Pendragon, the Head Dragon. Feel the flames revolving around your head, like a coronet of most holy light. That is your higher dragon essence, rising from your heart and dancing in a ring of ecstasy through and around your higher chakras.

Now see a writhing dragon in the flames under your feet, where you placed your torch. This is your lower dragon, the dragon of your dark, limited, unlit self, and it will writhe in pain until you deliver it from suf-fering by striking it through with your golden lance, your heavenly self which is contained in the dancing dragon of the supernal heights that gyrates around you.

Reach into your deepest heart, your highest dragon essence, and bring forth the golden lance, the ramrod of light that glances and flashes with divine fire, the inconceivable fire of Goddess-God that only your most exalted vision can delineate.

Plunge this lance into the dragon at your feet.

The lower dragon ceases its anguished writhing, and, charged with the dynamic energy of the higher dragon, begins to spiral upward in coils of light. It meets the Pendragon, and both enter a balletic sequence of supreme joy. The higher and the lower dragon merge in the Pendragon's pure golden light.

This is your heart-light. It is pulsating love, the love which creates, informs and sustains the universe.

You and your higher dragon are one; the higher dragon has absorbed the lower dragon.

After a minute or so, let the dragons disappear into the furnace, and the furnace disappear into the light of the star. Let the star recede until it becomes again the radiant jewel in your heart-centre.

Thank Archangel Michael for his protection and blessing, and end the ceremony by sealing your chakras.

When you are ready to do so (this may not be on the same day as you performed the first ceremony), implement the second ceremony. It is the same as the first, except that, instead of Archangel Michael, you call on the bright angel Brigid to oversee the inner working that you will undertake. Brigid ('brightness' or 'incandescence') is the feminine aspect of the great Christ being. She has an identity beyond that of the angels; but it is her angelic essence we call on for this ceremony, simply because, as angel healers, we are concerned with the focus of angelic cooperation.

You will need to essay both ceremonies many times over before the release of all the dross you have accumulated through-out many lives has been consumed. It is well worth the effort, however. Your subtle bodies will thrill with sensitive response to the spiritual currents of life, and their colours and forces will spring into fountains of pure and clear life and consciousness. 'Thus,' say the angels, 'men and women may answer to their angel selves, which are ever calling them to lives of purity, of high endeavour, and of joy.'

Concerning this ceremony, the angels tell us: 'The energies and presences which constitute the inner fire of the universe stand ready to release the forces of their element at humanity's bidding [for instance, whenever you wish to undergo the fire-cleansing ceremony], so that they may return to those days of pristine purity when angels walked with men.'

The angels also say that when we have become practised in the art of summoning the heavenly fire, we 'may learn to release the fiery energy and its guardians into the dark and noisome places of the earth, to drive away the evil atmosphere which humanity itself has created'. This skill will serve us well, there-fore, in the necessary work of space clearing, which, as angel healers, we must include in our essential repertoire.

Angel Raphael

Raphael, one of the great archangels, is associated with our throat chakra. In one sense, he has two aspects, because the top and the bottom of our spine – the essence of our 'tree of life', and the magical sword and lance within us – are linked with his influences. In one guise he appears as Saturn, ruler of the base of the spine and its chakra, whose colour is red. Saturn (who has been called 'Satan' – most unjustly, I feel!) is ancient, white-locked Father Time, the grim reaper who sets us our karmic lessons and trials, and holds us in imprisonment (in school!) until we have attained our 'degree'. Only then may we leave our academy of learning (earthly life) and escape into the freedom of the spirit.

But behind Father Saturn's stern exterior beats a golden heart, and in his austere eyes, if we observe carefully, a distinct twinkle is alight! He is truly Father Christmas, the red-robed guardian of the Festival of the Light, who comes out of the land of ethical ice and snow where Saturn lives (the barren, frozen, Arctic wilderness, steeped in night, which is a symbol of life lived without the genial and fecundating potency of the spirit), bringing us good cheer and the bountiful gifts which our successful schooling has attracted to us. We should never fear Father Saturn. There is no doubt whatsoever that this great being is filled with a tender, paternal love for us, even though his narrow gorges and straitened ways seem so daunting, harsh and dreary as by his dictates we pass along and through them. This is his domain, the hard and bitter aspect of life which no-one enjoys. (It has always intrigued me, as a herbalist, to note that it is often the very bitterest of herbs that dispense the greatest healing power!)

Saturn's labour is dirty work, but, after all, someone among the celestial company has to do it. And Saturn would always remind us that for every seemingly cruel experience which life can deal us, there is angelic healing and comfort, a gentle, sustaining touch from Nature, and spiritual succour from the wise ascended ones, if only we could always be persuaded to call on it and accept it.

There is a reflection of the great healer, Raphael, in this dispenser of bitter herbs whom we call Saturn. He is Raphael's essence as we perceive him at the start of our journey – ancient and burdened with years. Strangely, the angels tell us that it is at the beginning of our journey that we manifest 'old age' (truly an illusion). As we tread the evolutionary highway of the spirit, we 'advance ever into the springtime of our youth', growing younger and younger.

Mercury rules the throat chakra, the young, mirthful golden boy who is the epitome of youth and the antithesis of Saturn. He is Saturn's true reflection, and, again, we find that he is associated with the angel Raphael. He is the laughing 'outlaw', who is free from the constraints and restrictions of Saturn's severe and numerous laws. He sits at the top of the 'tree of life' (our spine) and joyfully leads us up into its crown, our own crown or head-centre, so that we become the Pendragon, the Head Dragon, the true personification of our own higher nature. Then he releases us into the stars, the spiritual heavens, where we receive the spiritual starlight and give it again from our heart-centre in a boundless pulsation of divine consciousness, which is love. This wonder we express in life by means of our head, our own globe or sphere or planet through which we articulate the quintessence of our higher nature – the mysterious, fiery dragon of the spirit, with its serpentine or wave motion that is supernal life, indeed all life, itself.

In his Saturnine guise, Raphael is Merlin, man of sorrows, he of bitter prophecy whose enchantments and potions bring resolution and healing through tears and 'madness' (genuine sanity juxtaposed against the 'norm' of insanity, and so falsely appearing to be madness). As Mercury, he is Robin Hood, spirit of the greenwood, who laughingly teaches us to live a simple, pure, exalted life, free from the laws that hamper, blind and corrupt; and instructs us in stealing from the rich to give to the poor.

A deep mystery is enshrined here. The whole motion of life is geared to this sacred and mighty principle – that the stronger force gives unstintingly to the weaker, that the rich give to the poor. The ignorance and foolishness of worldly values blocks this law, so that congestive heart failure (of our civilization) is the result. We need our hero, Robin Hood, and of course Maid Marian, without whom his mission would not be possible, to save us! Robin Hood reflects Jesus, another 'outlaw' of his own time, who taught us a new system of values and who had his other half, his own feminine 'double M' by his side. Are we beginning to get a glimpse of who Raphael truly is?

Raphael is she-he who, through his guardianship as alpha and omega of the spine – which is both our sword and our lance that connects the two, serving as a lightning-rod for heaven – unites heaven and earth within the dimensions of his vision, purpose and power, so revealing him as the glorious angel of the Holy Grail. It was his great healing mission to work with Jesus and Mary Magdalene, the two aspects, masculine and feminine, of the great Christ Being in the heavens who sought to descend to earth through them. And how could this be otherwise, when Jesus and Mary themselves brought forth the Holy Grail, the divine connection between heaven and earth that will be restored to this generation, our own, who currently walks the earth? As the Angel of the Grail who bears its healing energies, Raphael's key word is 'Consolamentum'. He speaks this word of measureless dimension through the mighty Angel of Music, the angel Israfel. It sounds from the higher atmosphere like a peal of clear bells from heaven, supernaturally sweet, yet borne forth in an undertone of cosmic grandeur. This word in itself can heal and soothe, and summon the magic of wholeness to the ailing, fragmented soul. It is the title of a secret ceremony administered by the Cathars of medieval France, whereby one of the *perfecti* (the Cathar priests) would bestow the Consolamentum on a member of their congregation once they had declared themselves ready to receive this special initiation and blessing. It is connected with the mysteries of the Holy Grail, and it is reported that many wonders were experienced, among them a clear and direct cognition of the spiritual worlds, whilst the ceremony was underway.

When we wish to become angel healers, we enter the school of Raphael and his company of healing angels, and we have to learn how to so connect earth and heaven within ourselves that we cannot help but usher the healing forces to those who stand in need of them. The next stage of our journey into knowledge of the great angel Raphael and his circle of angels is to enter into meditation, using the techniques we have learned concerning withdrawing into the heart, wherein lies the star and the rose (our heart of hearts), so that our 'mind in the heart' springs into unalloyed consciousness, and our imagination becomes a powerful tool of vision, a creator of worlds.

We might even see our imagination actually becoming the shining angel Samandiriel herself, she of the Divine Fruits of Celestial Vision, who, 'clad in the beauty of a thousand stars', leaves a bright trail of manifestation in her wake as she leads us into the sublime light of our deepest dreams.

Raphael and his Company of Healing Angels

Sit with the star of spiritual light shining above you, and focus gently on your breathing. Breathe in the light of the spiritual star, and breathe it out as a gift to the world.

Contemplate the greatness and the mystery of the archangel Raphael, She-He who is the Angel of the Holy Grail and the guardian of the secret of the spine, which is our stairway to heaven. All healing flows forth from Raphael. He shepherds this healing force as it radiates from the Golden One, the heavenly being whom some call Christ-Brigid.

It is time go deeper into meditation. Listen with your inner ears to the sound that is coming to you from the higher spheres...

The archangel Raphael is calling you into his presence. Let your inner eyes open to the glory of his manifestation in the spiritual worlds.

His form is mighty, as tall as a cathedral. His eyes shine

with loving compassion, emitting a great light, and yet they are as mellow and gentle and deep as the glow of ancient and mysterious gold. His melodious mouth utters rhythmic healing chants, beautiful in their vibration, becoming from time to time a great burst of exquisite song which pierces the listening soul with an irresistible tide of love as renewal, as reawakening, as revivification.

Hear his soft chanting and his burst of song through which the cadence of the word 'Consolamentum' beats like a spirit drum, and feel all your energies in all your bodies — mind, emotion, soul and physical — rise as if newborn from an ocean of sparkling drops of the utmost purity, rise in white garments to the blazing disc of the morning sun.

Rest in that perfect light, fresh and revitalized, created anew.

There is the fragrance of cleansing joy in the robes of Raphael, and golden healing in his wings. Those golden wings of light enfold you in their great arcs of sweeping spiritual force, and you know yourself as perfect in light, perfect, perfect within the sunlight of his healing embrace.

Now see his vast host of healing angels as they come in countless choirs to the golden-winged feet of their master, ready to receive his blessing and the touch of his radiant hands, which bestow the gift of spiritual life-forces from the ineffable and cosmic reservoir that is his very being.

Some come on his own golden and yellow ray, bright and deep in hue, some gently glowing as with the marigold light of a summer evening sun, some with the celandine light of the early morning rays.

Some come in on a single colour ray, all blending in an assembled mystery of soft rose, or glowing emerald-green, or sweet heavenly blue.

Some sweep in like a tide, arrayed in iridescent rainbow colours, subtle, shimmering and beautiful, as though their hues shone through the purest crystal.

Some bear a most holy pearlescent light which is wonderful to see: the pearly light of unicorns from the high places of the soul, and of precious stones from a sublime sea that beats on the shores of paradise.

A great host of the healing angels is dressed in simple garments of the purest white, an unearthly whiteness which is so vast and deep that it is the heart of peace itself, making earthly whiteness seem almost dark in comparison, and yet you note how soft and gentle to the eye is the whiteness of these sacred garments, a whiteness that does not dazzle, as if pushing away, but rather tenderly enfolds you in its magical light.

The song from Raphael's lips becomes speech. 'Come to me, all who are sick, who are weary, who are burdened of heart and full of sorrow and pain, and you shall be made whole.'

The hosts of healing angels carry you into the heart of Archangel Raphael.

Here all is still. His healing chants, joyous song and comforting words have become a golden silence. Listen to the healing wisdom of that silence. Feel and absorb its tremendous power. Rest in its hushed, encompassing stillness.

Take some moments to enjoy this utter stillness and its healing balm of peace.

Before you, in your heart's vision, descends a simple

white staff. Around it, to the left, twines a golden serpent. On the right, its twin curls around the staff in a similar ascending spiral. The handle of the staff is winged. It is the caduceus.

'Take my staff, and wield it,' says the voice of Archangel Raphael.

The scene changes. You find yourself upon a road, winding into the distance. At your side stands Merlin. He wears hermit's robes and a pilgrim's hat. He bears the caduceus, and now he places it in your right hand, and a vial of healing ointment in your left. You understand that the caduceus is a gift from the king of heaven and earth, given to you through Archangel Raphael, and that the healing ointment is a gift from the queen of earth and heaven, given to you by her devoted servant, Merlin.

Merlin speaks. There is a kindly light in his eye. 'Become the Divine Physician. Let the angelic healing forces flow through your heart and your hands,' Merlin says to you.

He raises his hand in blessing. 'I give you the most holy benediction of She who is Hidden,' he says, and places his hand on the crown of your head. You feel the benediction coursing through you like the fire of the sun and the fire of the moon. He turns you around to face the sun, and sets your feet upon the Path.

Gently emerge from your meditation, and seal your centres (crown, mid-brow, throat, heart, solar plexus) with the brilliant silver cross contained in a ring of light.

Meeting Merlin

To enter more deeply into the mysteries of Archangel Raphael, we need to explore those aspects of him which are the living dynamic of Merlin and of Robin Hood. Both of these figures, who are legendary but who manifested in human form in Britain, Merlin in the 6th century and Robin at the time of the Crusades, are the human guise of great godly beings. Merlin was, of course, King Arthur's mentor and guardian, a prophet and Druid enchanter of high degree. He led King Arthur to the secret queen who presented him with the sacred sword Excalibur, the Sword of Safekeeping for the nation which would preserve the Holy Grail and give its essence to the world in the next age (today).

Robin of the Greenwood was the outlaw who, on returning from the Crusades, found that Britain, the holy isle, fell short of upholding faithful Templar values, the values and principles of what Robin had been taught comprised the true Way that the Christ Being had demonstrated and revealed to humanity. Robin, a member of the Knights Templar, gathered his followers around him and lived in profound intimacy with nature, following a life of moral nobility deep in the spiritually nurturing greenwood that was true to the spiritual code he had learned from his esoteric order of knights.

As healers, we need to attune to and understand something of Merlin and Robin's magic and wildness, for Merlin was a forest dweller too, forsaking all earthly comforts to dwell in the great Caledonian forest. This harmony with nature, with the spirits that ensoul her and the healing magic that she secretes in her heart, is precisely what, to its great detriment, orthodox medicine has lost sight of, treating us as if we belonged to a universe alienated from nature and the spirit. We cannot despise the source of wisdom, which lies in nature and in the spirit, and expect to prosper. One day, Archangel Raphael and our medical establishments will work together consciously, and the result will flood the world with a stupendous healing power.

Meeting Merlin

Create the six-pointed star in your heart, and breathe in its light. Focus on your breath's rise and fall, and how the in-breath draws the light into the farthest fathoms of your being, and the out-breath sends it forth across the world.

You are sleeping in your bed. It is deepest night. Touch that level of profound rest and quietness that peaceful sleep brings to you.

Suddenly, a gentle whisper rouses you. You awake fully. Your fairy ally, a beautiful, evolved being who moves in swirls of amethyst and rose mist, is standing at your bedside, smiling down at you.

You feel her angelic essence, but you know that she is one of the noble fairy folk: a nature spirit. She is your mirror, your twin in Faery Land, who protects you.

You wonder if in fact you have been transported into Faery Land, and look around the room. It is your own familiar room, just as it always is during the night hours. The fairy being at your side makes a motion with her slim white arm, and you see an arched, oaken door appear in the very centre of the room. It is exquis-itely carved with mystic symbols and wise ancient faces of ageless beauty.

The door begins to swing open. Magically, there beyond the door is an enchanted woodland, lit by stars and a great, round, full moon, bright as a miracle.

'Come to the fairy revels,' says your companion.

She takes you by the hand and you rise from your bed and walk out into the mysterious woodland. Soft musk scent rises from the shadowed ground like a secret, thrilling benediction, and the trees, in full leaf, surround you like mighty guardians, steadfast and benevolent.

You see a muted, glimmering light ahead, and suddenly you step into a wide moonlit glade. The flickering light you saw shines from a golden lantern which hangs at the entrance to a cave, overhung with ferns and twining plants.

At the entrance to the cave, a majestic old man, robed in hermit's garb and with flowing, snow-white hair, stands with one hand upon a great staff.

You see that the staff is the caduceus, a rod formed from two intertwining serpents. Over the old man's dark robes a light of pure gold moves and shimmers like fairy dust, starry and magical as the muted fire of the stars. As you watch, you realize that the moving light is a great golden dragon that coils and spirals around him in serpentine motion. This is Merlin, Chief Druid; Merlin, the Magician; Merlin, Prince of Enchanters.

'I am the Keeper of the Sacred Law. I am the Keeper of the Eternal Secret,' he says to you.

He lifts his staff, and suddenly the moonlit glade bursts into colour and life. Troupes of fairies pour into it from between the trees, some descending from the treetops. Some mysteriously appear, as if from the depths of the ground. Fairy lights shine from the tree branches, bright and vivid yet tender too, soft and warm. Their colours are a pure delight, a supernatural festival of rose and crimson, yellow and marigold and peach, orange and blue, gold and lilac, violet, green, indigo, silver, ruby, sky blue and dusk blue, turquoise, amethyst, amber and glistening pearl, all showering their enchanting rays about you so that you are bathing in a thousand converging rivers of colour.

'Dance with the fairies. Fill your heart with fairy delight,' says Merlin.

In an instant the fairies form a great ring about you and whirl you off into a joyful, exhilarating dance, wild as the spirit of nature. Dance, dance with the fairies, and know that you dance with the stars and the planets, that your dance is the dance of worlds within worlds, eternally, ecstatically turning. Dance with the immortals, the ever-young, and bring forth your angelic and your fairy self.

How beautiful, how intriguing, how mysterious the forms of the fairies are as they flash in the light of the moon and the stars and the happy lantern colours. You become aware of Merlin, nodding and smiling beyond the circle, and yet he seems to lead the dance from the centre.

You look keenly into the middle of the circle. You are aware of a dimensionless point, a hallowed void – the sacred no-thing around which the components of each atom dance...

You find, in the joy of the dance, that you are growing quite philosophical. You know that it is because your heart is connected to Merlin and his radialling fairy forces.

You see that this Fairy Dance is the dance of the struc-ture of the atom, and that atoms are mandalas. 'The mandala is the innermost pattern of creation,' Merlin tells you in silent thought-communion. 'They are pictures of the sacred dance of life, the whirling dervishes. The energy dance around the centre of the atom is a dance around a void – a mystic centre which is non-manifest in the material world. If we enlarged the size of an atom to that of a planet, its nucleus, the centre, would still be smaller than a pinhead. Yet everything revolves around this sanctified heart, this holy no-thing.'

Merlin smiles, and shows you the great trick of the fairies: how they can be minuscule or instantly grow to a size much bigger than ourselves. 'Theirs is the gift of the centre, which knows that force is real and form is not,' he explains.

You continue to revel in the Fairy Dance as Merlin speaks again. 'Have not your scientists only recently discovered that there are twelve subatomic particles?' he asks. 'Of course there are! Twelve planets to our solar system, dancing around the sacred centre of inconceivable fire, twelve revolving constellations that make up the zodiac, twelve Knights of the Round Table that surround King Arthur, twelve great labours of Hercules, the soul of humanity; and twelve disciples that form the blessed circle around the Christ Being. Has not organized religion, and later the orthodoxy of science and the pall of materialism, deprived and robbed you of your love of the fairies and the fairy worlds? Take it back, my friend. Take this power back into your heart through the Fairy Dance. It is the dance of your soul around your spirit. Reclaim this blessed power, dear healer. You cannot advance without it; and with it you will bring your world into a harmony that is the star of your deepest dreams and which burns beyond even your highest hopes.'

With a far-flung joy that encompasses the heavens and the earth, and your being that circles between the two, you take back into your heart the love of the spirit of nature and her magical laughing people that the human world has tried to hide from you. You know that now you are whole again, and that Merlin's lesson is complete.

As Merlin's lesson ends, the fairies release you from the whirling crescendo of the dance. You find yourself standing before the great sage of spiritual law, his student and his friend. You are known to Merlin now, and he smiles on and blesses your healing aspirations. You sense Archangel Raphael in the depths of his eyes, and your heart-mind knows that his company of healing angels dances around Merlin with a reverence that is almost worship. On impulse, you kneel to this stern and kindly ancient.

He raises you by the hand, and by the hand he leads you into the depths of his cave, before which, in the moon-enchanted glade, the fairy revels took place.

You gaze around in rapture. Deep within, the cave is composed of myriads of crystals, scintillating with every gorgeous tint and hue, some of which are not colours that are seen on earth. Through this living wonder you go, and find yourself at another doorway of the cave, overlooking a deep, still, clear forest pool.

Merlin stands behind you, and draws you into his heart. He has become a great tree, a mighty, steadfast oak, whose branches shelter and enfold you.

How utterly supported, how safe and deeply rooted into the good firm earth you feel, as you rest peacefully in the protective heart of Merlin.

'Child of Earth,' Merlin says to you, in a voice as hushed and deep as the ocean. 'Come to me, rest in my heart as you do now, whenever you need wisdom, whenever you need vision, whenever you need fairy contact, whenever you need succour, whenever you need to renew your healing forces, whenever you need peace.'

As Merlin speaks, the sun rises and makes an angelic glory on the surface of the clear, still forest pool. Merlin, the oak tree, also lights up from within, and casts a glory and a mystery of radiant colour into the waters of the pool, until they are aflame in a cascading flood of morning's purest light.

'This is the glory of the New Day for humanity that is already dawning,' Merlin says to you. 'You have an important part to play. Never forget it. I am always here to help you. This is my divine mission for the unfolding age. May your soul be as clear, as radiant, as many-coloured, as restful and as deep as this sacred pool.'

You rest easily within Merlin, looking out in wonder at the great expanse of water, filled with the magnificence, the flame, the beatitude, of the noble dawn.

When you are ready, call your fairy ally to you, and let her tenderly escort you to the door that leads into your bedroom. This is done in a moment. Get into bed, and feel yourself sinking down into present everyday reality as your fairy ally creates symbols of blessing over your recumbent form.

Firmly touch down, seal your centres, and, because you have been to Faery Land, gently stamp both feet.

The Fairy Lover

Now we progress from grave ancient to golden youth! It is important to contain both Merlin and Robin in our hearts, because it is at the centrepoint, the heart (which is also the apex, or the highest point of our consciousness), that they meet and are one. When within us the wisdom of the earth (Merlin-Saturn) meets the consciousness of the spirit (Robin-Mercury), the antahkarana, the rainbow bridge, springs into being.

It is most interesting that in fairy lore, the leprechaun, a little old man who is a way-shower for the human soul, as he indicates by cobbling magical shoes, is deeply associated with Merlin (you might say they are his little clones!), and that wherever the leprechaun was seen by country people, such a place either originally was, or became, the site of rainbows and natural springs. Mercury or Robin, the messenger of the sun, represents the rays that create the rainbow and cause the springing forth of all creation. The great rainbow bridge that Merlin and Robin create together is that bridge between spirit and soul which connects our earthly self with the glorious light, seven-rayed, of the Divine. When we walk over the rainbow bridge into the golden world of the spirit, not in death but in full consciousness as we actually live out our earthly lives, we walk into freedom and limitlessness. This is the realm that the angels share with us, the source from which we give healing.

The idea of the following guided visualization is to recognize within ourselves the sacred marriage of the spirit and the soul that creates the rainbow bridge. It is given here as Maid Marian journeying to meet Robin, but please mix and match according to your perspective!

The Sacred Marriage

Sit upright, your spine supported if necessary, and ensure that you are comfortable and relaxed. Focus on your heart-centre and breathe gently, easily and slowly. In your mind's eye, let your heart be as a jewel or a crystal into which you are gazing.

You are standing beneath the boughs of a tree in a forest at the breaking of a summer dawn.

Murmurs of birdsong sound in the still, cool air, a sweet liquid piping and fluting as if from far, far above, as though it echoed in the grand, solemn space of a cathedral. The silver-grey light of the early morning has a rapt, enthralled quality, like a beating heart in a lover's expectant breast.

The rays of the rising sun smile suddenly over the waiting forest, and all is transformed. The birdsong becomes a mighty chorus of joy; you listen and watch in rapture as small woodland animals appear in the forest glade before you, intent upon the business of the morning. They are unafraid, showing only curiosity and friendliness as you turn your gaze on them.

With you, they are aware of the presence of the Great Spirit and, with you, they offer thanksgiving for the birth of this perfect day.

You are wearing a leaf-green gown, as if composed from the newborn sunlight and the viridian green of springtime leaves. You notice that there are translucent jewels sewn into your clothing which catch the light in dancing flashes and simultaneously give it forth again in shades of their own mystic brilliance.

On your feet are soft shoes made from cloth of gold. The threads in them shine in the sunbeams, and as you begin to walk deeper into the singing forest it is as if every step you take can heal and bless the earth with sacred gold from the heart of the sun.

You realize that you have been given these shoes to tread softly upon the Earth, to revere and worship her with an offering of your human love, for verily she is a loving, living Goddess.

You press on deeper and deeper into the forest because

your true love awaits you, the pure-hearted warrior who is the mirror of your eternal self. Every step you take is one of jubilance and wonder, your heart alight with the promise, the anticipation, of his waiting presence. You listen to the birdsong, you taste and smell the clean, fresh, vigorous scents of the woodland, you see the sunlight dancing on the leaves and the forest floor, and the sapphire vault of the skies rolling like a blue carpet of peace over all the world.

It occurs to you that all creation is dancing with Goddess and that it would be good for you to dance too. You dance there in a shining glade among the trees, lightly, airily, like a spirit of nature, and it seems to you in your joy as if you danced with the scintillating stars and all the turning firmament. As your dance ends, you are aware that its sacred configurations has brought someone — the pulse of your life — into your company.

You approach an ancient and majestic tree whose great arching branches create a quiet green sanctuary, flourishing with mistletoe and sunlit leaves. Here Robin, the Hooded Man, awaits.

Robin is smiling, rapt at your approach. He is tall, keen-eyed, supple with youth and beauty, yet old as the stars. He enfolds you in an embrace of warmth and love and the protection he brings as warrior of the soul.

As for a moment your body and your being fuse with his and you become as one, you sense in the love between you the strength and the essence of the mighty prehensile roots of the oak-temple, coiling away from the huge bole of the tree with serpentine dignity, outstretching in the darkness to the sacred core of Mother Earth. Breathing and seeing with you, Robin accompanies you as you walk side by side along the path that the western roots follow underground.

You come to a secret cave, overhung with ivy and scrolls of fern. Hand in hand, you and Robin, united spirit of the greenwood, enter in.

The cave is dim and vast, whispering with echoing murmurs from far away. It is lit by a single soft golden flame, burning candlelike in a fissure of the rock which stands as a pillar at the centre of the cave. Around this immense pillar lie 12 sleeping knights, their armour shining like the white spume of the sea. They form a ring of light around the great king, Arthur, who sleeps on a dais in the midst of them; magically, you and Robin are drawn into his dream, the sacred dream of King Arthur in which he is steeped until the time shall come for him and his white knights to awake.

The dream of King Arthur is the form and essence of a mystic rose, mellifluently pink as a warm summer sunrise. This gentle emanation of colour is a magical power flowing forth from the heart of the king, and the heart of the king is the rose, a temple of exquisite form and fragrance that you and Robin can enter together, to kneel at the golden altar there.

Awake in his dream, the king smiles on you and Robin, and pronounces a blessing over you as you kneel together in the beautiful temple of the rose. You and your soul-warrior are made one, for when you rise you are wed.

In the brilliance shed from the glory of this moment, you see clearly that the mystic rose is blooming in your heart and in Robin's heart.

In joy, you breathe deeply of the fragrance of the rose,

and the knowledge comes to you that King Arthur is present in the soul of the Earth, that he is the guardian of Britain, and that all divine guardians of other lands are also present in Britain's soul, in those refined spheres behind the physical life which some call the Dreamtime; and you know that as King Arthur sleeps he guards the sacred rose, the rose which is the heart of all things and also your own heart, the fountain of renewal for all the world.

You and Robin drink deeply of this magical and blessed fountain, for you find that you can indeed drink in this divine essence.

When you are refreshed and made new, you find that you are kneeling together beneath the boughs of the oak-temple, alone again with Robin in the peace and beauty of the forest.

You and Robin are one, and you are forever bonded with his laughing, dancing, eternally young spirit which enshrines all the spiritual secrets of nature.

As you reach out to touch the wise and ancient oak tree, you receive a blessing from Merlin, the great seer, and beyond him from some omnipotent entity that you can only conceive of as the Queen of the Stars. Accept the blessing; absorb it.

You know that King Arthur, Merlin, Robin, and you yourself, are all this mighty queen's spiritual children; and that Merlin will keep her mysteries hidden until the time is right for their disclosure.

The forest, its wonder, its secrets, its enchanted people, recedes within you, enfolded by the petals of the rose in your heart. Come back gently, touch down in the mundane world, and carry these treasures within you.

Seal your centres with the bright silver cross in a ring of light and affirm:

I bring my mind, my emotions, every thought arising within me, together into the presence of divine healing.

I receive the blessing of peace into my deepest heart.

I breathe forth this peace into the heart of the world as living light which is the radiance of peace and spiritual healing.

I find ways to express peaceful living and the blessing of angel healing in my community.

The final lap of our journey into the mysteries of Raphael now awaits us. It concerns the great enigma of the Holy Grail, and a message for all those who read these words and aspire to become healers who work with angels.

The Holy Grail is coming to us, and will soon be with us. Its wonders will be given to those who walk the earth today. The angels are asking us to make every effort to prepare for this inconceivable illumination and initiation, because those of us who have consciously drawn close to the angels and who seek to cooperate with them in their work for humanity will be the first to accept the initiation of the Holy Grail. It will therefore be our privileged responsibility to help others to realize the importance of also accepting its gifts in initiation, and to encourage them to feel sufficiently confident and motivated to do so.

Djwhal Khul, the Tibetan master who inspired Alice Bailey to write 25 books on esotericism, predicted that hundreds of thousands will take this initiation. Let us be daring, and entertain the hope that *millions* will take it! The angels assure us that such a hope is by no means in vain.

Margaret Bailey and I can hint at a few of the secrets of the Grail, even before it is retrieved. (Its location, history, and how we will receive its virtues are the subject of our forthcoming book.) The cup that it represents is a vast spiritual cup, a cosmic cup of recipience in which we are all united as one – every kingdom, from nature and her spirits through humanity to the angels – every member of every kingdom is united and as one in the divine receptacle of the Grail cup. We have received indications that although an actual cup will be found, the Grail is by no means a physical cup. Something stupendous will also be unearthed, and it will reveal to us the secret of ascension whilst we are still here on earth.

Meditation, art, prayer – all these things provide a method for us to enter heaven whilst we are still attached to our physical bodies. But the Grail will give to every soul who receives it into their heart a method of ascension which so far in the history of the earth has only been available to the highest of the adepts; and it will 'rend in two' the veil of the temple, that which hangs between us and divine vision so that when we touch down after meditation, the pall of earthliness which drains the magic out of life soon reasserts itself and makes things seem dreary and difficult again! That obscuring veil will go, and we shall know heaven whilst we walk the earth. Once this new consciousness has been established, it will be the start of everything. The great emancipation of the human soul, with all its magnificent horizons and its transformation of life on earth, will be underway.

How can we prepare for the coming of the Grail? Follow the star in your heart, the star of the spirit! Lessen the claims of earthliness and materialism, and devote some time each day to meditation, angel communion, invocation, prayer and purification. These simple, gentle methods will throw off the chains that presently bind us, and allow an impersonal love for all to flow freely. Become familiar with the star and the rose, with the sanctity of silence, with magical breathing and giving forth the light. Purify yourself and your environment, using the methods given, and diligently train yourself in the art of angel healing, if that is your chosen path. The angels tell us that we cannot yet encompass with our everyday minds what is meant by 'angel healing'. We tend to think in terms of disease and pain manifesting through physical maladies, and of course these problems comprise a part of its compass; but they are not the whole. We will give forth healing in cooperation with the angels in ways we have never dreamed in the days to come. The ethers and the thought-spheres of our world are desperately in need of decontamination and of healing. The Grail is the spearhead of this planetary transfiguration, and it is this for which we now prepare.

Several thousand years ago, we managed to lose the Grail and drive its perfection from our consciousness and our world. The Christed couple, Jesus and Mary Magdalene, retrieved it for us by dint of unconscionable sacrifice inspired by a wondrous love for humanity – for humanity as a whole and for each individual member. It was the point of their entire mission, because the divine alchemy of the Grail is the teaching of 'the Way', which they revealed to us in greater radiance and dimension than it had ever been revealed before. If we do not follow the Way, we cannot receive the inestimable gifts of the Grail. More and more people today are becoming disenchanted with the lure of selfishness and materialism and the denial of love, harmony and kindness which following it entails. These people, turning from the call of the darkness, tread the path which is the Way, be they agnostics, atheists, new agers, pagans, naturists or members of the world's orthodox religions. The Way is not a religion – it is the Way! Sufficient numbers are now on this divine path for the Grail to be given to humanity; and it will be given.

What we need to understand is that the Grail has been preserved for us by the angelic and fairy streams of life. If we say it baldly – that the angels and the fairies have kept safe the Holy Grail for us – we may imagine the derisive laughter that our statement would invoke from many people. This in itself is remarkable evidence of the conditioning and programming that we have received through the ages from those adversary forces who sought to create a mindset in us that would deny the very

existence of what would set us free – for the adversary forces
receive the benefits of our enslavement. Nature mysticism, a
love of the angels and the fairies, are precisely what nourish the
sacred Grail forces. These forces are what set us free as spiritual
beings and release the powers of the spirit through the shining
rainbow of the soul, so connecting us with the seven-rayed
potency of the Divine. Perhaps we can see now why the authority of earthly establishments, who love to control us, have always
taught us to mock the idea of fairies and angels and the Holy
Grail, and to alienate ourselves from nature.

The following guided visualization gives an idea of how the
angels and the fairies work together to sustain the Grail energies.
The human Grail – our divine inheritance of the powers of the
soul and the unspeakable privilege of living in heaven whilst we
walk the earth – has been lost to us, stolen from us in ages past
by our own wanton foolishness. It is this paradise that we shall
regain. If the Angel Grail had not been maintained for us and
our world, earth would have ceased to exist by now as a life-
bearing planet. (The quotes in the following text are the words
of Geoffrey Hodson. This great angel seer refers to the Sun Spirit
as 'He', but there can be no doubt that this Being is a perfect
expression of both the Sacred Feminine and the Sacred
Masculine principles – Christ-Brigid, or, as John the Beloved
Disciple explains, 'the Spirit and the Bride'.)

The Angel Grail

Begin to breathe quietly through the heart-centre,
creating the form of the shining star there as a six-
pointed radiance and seeing its rays envelop you from
that sacred central point within your being.

It is midsummer eve, night of magic and revelation.
All through the fairy worlds, the angels are gathering
together those nature spirits who are ready to enter
into the angelic line of evolution. Everywhere there is

festivity and a sense of the grandeur of the occasion. At this time, a great ritual of communion with and worship of the sun is enacted by the angelic hosts.

The fairies share this joyful communion, and their revels on midsummer eve are touched by a dusting of the deepest spiritual magic, embraced and nurtured by a secret quality in the moonlight and the radiance of the stars through which they weave their merry dances.

The angels assemble at the higher altitudes above all this merrymaking. Their delight is as keen as that of the fairies, but it also sounds a note of deeper, sublime joy, as though a sonorous cathedral organ intermingles with the silvery sweetness of pealing bells. The angels form circles according to their hierarchical degrees which rise, tier upon tier, as a magnificent living structure that reaches into worlds beyond worlds. 'The radiant bodies of the shining ones thus united form a chalice of living light.'

This great sacramental cup reaches from the lowest level of the earth, where the fairies sport and play, to the jewel of the spirit that is the sun. Every atom of aspiration which comprises the angelic hosts strives upward to the sun. 'Every heart is full of love and adoration; every eye turned upwards to the Lord of Life. The auric forces are all blended to make a perfect whole... thus the cup is formed.'

As the chalice appears, the adoration of the angels creates a river of many colours which streams upwards, heaven bound, through the channel of the cup created by their thoughts and their ethereal bodies, so that it springs as a fountain of exaltation until it reaches the higher angels, who unite their limitless love and aspiration to the rising current, which becomes a great torrent and rises to the mighty archangels, who receive it and usher it into the heart of the sun. There it enters the being of the 'great and nameless One who is the Spirit of the Sun and the Lord of Power and Life in every world'.

A burst of music fills the aerial heights. The reverence and prayer of the angels has attained such a height that it must now be expressed in the dynamic of music, because it has become a part of the creative force itself. Its glory is a swell of sound and shining light. 'Adoration flows forth as from a single heart. A living ecstasy pervades the soul of every angel devotee. Wave upon wave of joy, of exaltation and of living light and sound, sweep through the angelic ranks.

'The light within the chalice grows more and more intense. Bright colours flash and play across its wide expanse. The upward-flowing force [from the chalice] lifts every angel into realms of being far above those in which it usually dwells. Each one is exalted into the presence of our Lord the Sun; every aura expands with solar light and power.

'All sense of time and space is lost. Still the flood of angel love and adoration flows towards the sun. Still, with wills united and hearts overflowing, they pour forth the very essence of their souls in uttermost surrender to their Lord. The music grows grander and more majestic. A mighty and harmonious volume of sound accompanies the worship of the angel hosts. In that music, every aspiration is fulfilled.

'At last the highest point is reached, the peak of ecstasy attained. The chalice is full formed in all its perfect beauty of colour, light and sound.

'At that moment, when at once the highest and the

deepest note is struck, the answer comes. The Spirit of the Sun pours forth His power in a flood of golden light. Formed of white fire at its core, and glowing with golden sunlight shot through with all the seven-fold colours of His rays, the power descends and enters every angel soul, filling it with life and light, until the lowest ring is reached. There it is held, whilst all drink deeply of the consecrated wine of solar life.

'The music ceases. Silence marks the consummation of the solemn Eucharist. A stillness most profound sur-rounds and pervades the solar rites. All angels meditate upon the glory now revealed within their inmost beings. All fall into a state of deepest contem-plation. Then, at last, music bursts forth once more in a glad paean of thanksgiving and of joy. Angel choirs take up the song, singing in vast multitudes around the throne of light...

'In the midst, our Lord the Sun Himself shines forth, golden and glowing in all His sevenfold beauty. His solar angels bow low in reverence before the majesty which He thus reveals. Of that Presence no tongue can tell, nor any words disclose Its splendour; even the highest angels bow down in utter veneration and silence before that awful Self-revealing.

'On every side the fields of space are filled with glory and with countless throngs of shining ones. And in the midst of them in all His splendour shines our Lord the Sun.

'Each angel sees the vision splendid in varying degree, according to the power of its perception and the stature to which it has attained. However great or small its soul may be, it is filled with the knowledge of the glory of the sun.

'Thousands who had not yet attained to individual existence pass into angelhood, leaving the days of their faeriedom behind. These are received with exceeding joy into the angels' ranks.

'The whole angelic evolution, down to the smallest nature spirit, has been illumined and blessed by the celebration of the mystery of the sun.'

Allow yourself to bathe in the glorious emanations of this sun ceremony. Hail your brethren, your fellows, your companions of your earthly and your heavenly life – the angels and the fairies.

Touch down gently, emerge from your meditation in your own time, and seal your centres.

Finally, after you have worked through the meditations and contemplations given in this chapter, dedicate yourself to the service of Archangel Raphael and his company of healing angels. Choose a time when you feel particularly attuned and receptive to angelic influences, and, in your own words, which will carry your special vibration and convey your soul to Archangel Raphael, conduct a little dedication ceremony.

Light a white candle, remembering to light it with the flame in your heart as well as with physical ignition. Tell Archangel Raphael all your hopes and aspirations relating to your development as an angel healer. Receive the dynamism of his potent blessing.

CHAPTER FIVE

THE HEALER'S TREASURY

There are a few further steps to take in developing the art of angel healing before we advance to its practical application, although of course the progress you make through individual effort, aspiration and experience will be the true measure of your qualification.

Space Clearing

It is always advisable to cleanse your surroundings, even when you intend only to meditate or to perfect your healing techniques. Before treating yourself or a patient (whether or not the patient is present or absent), the process is indispensable.

No great effort is required for everyday space clearing. You can simply:

- call on the Cleansing Angel Vwyamus (see Chapter One);
- employ the method of the Violet Flame (see Chapter One);
- use the idea of the sun ceremony described at the end of Chapter Four to invoke that great, glorious presence of the Sun Being, Christ-Brigid, praying that Her-His benign Presence will transmute all

shadows and negative energy into sparkling, high-spin, angel-touched atoms;

- call on the angels generally to purify your environment with the cleansing flames of spirit fire;

- imagine a great, crested, rolling wave of a spiritual sea sweeping through the room and onward, taking with it in its crashing, rotating cylinder all undesirable influence and energy.

These methods are for general cleansing purposes. However, you may encounter situations where an atmosphere is very poisonous at the psychic level. Clearing this energy is part of your work as an angel healer, but it is very important that you proceed with caution. Bear these rules in mind.

1   Sit down quietly by yourself, and, with both feet resting firmly on the ground, call on the power of the sun.

2   Create the form of a great silver cross contained within a ring of light, and place yourself and any who are with you in its centre.

3   Call on the protection of your guardian angel, and then of Archangel Michael, the Protector. Ask him to monitor the entire cleansing procedure.

4   Ask Archangel Michael if it is right for you to proceed alone. Communicate through your heart-centre.

5   Wait patiently for Michael's answer. It will be given through the medium of your will. If you feel encouraged to go ahead, it is safe to do so. If you feel any obstruction or inhibition at the level of your will concerning the implementation of the cleansing process, you must not put it into practice. You could either endanger yourself or another (perhaps someone living in the astral dimensions of life).

Another method of receiving Archangel Michael's instructions is to visualize a set of traffic lights. See the three vertical discs unlit. Watch as one lights up. If the amber light starts to glow, its message is that you may go ahead, but the present time is ill-auspiced. Choose another day to carry out your cleansing ritual.

If Archangel Michael advises against the procedure, there are four stumbling blocks which are the most probable reasons for his warning.

1   A trapped human soul is causing the energy disturbance, and would suffer as the result of an attempt at space clearing.

If this is the case, summon the Healing Angels and place the matter in their hands; then call on the angel Colopatiron, the angel who frees us from imprisonment, to lend his assistance to the situation. It is also important to create the star in your heart, and gently enfold the struggling, confused soul in its light. Send them the fragrance of the mystic rose. Request the protection of the angels throughout. Ask for Archangel Michael's instructions regarding the relevant space clearing again after three days, and see if his answer has changed.

If not, repeat the process outlined above, including the creation of the rainbow bridge, which you can then invite the distressed soul to cross.

If none of this has any effect (which will be very rare), continue to hold the situation in your spiritual heart-light each day (just take a short moment) and instruct the angels to stand by so that they may continue to give assistance as the dark energy begins to loose its grip. You will know when to return to

the task, if it still requires your attention, because
the angels will alert you through your intuition.

2 An unpleasant entity is the cause of the problem,
   which should not be tackled alone; therefore it will
   be necessary to form a small group. Follow the
   instructions for the Cleansing Ritual below.

3 The etheric conditions are so poisonous that group
   effort is required to alleviate the problem.
   Attempting to deal with the situation alone could
   overwhelm you or cause you to be unwell. Use the
   method outlined in the Cleansing Ritual below.

4 Distorted earth forces are present which require the
   attention of an expert.
      If the earth forces are constricted, choked, or
   distorted, you will need to contact an earth healer. If
   this is not possible, call on Archangel Raphael and
   the healing angels and ask them to form a circle of
   healing and protection around the affected area.
   Then summon the great Angel Sandalphon, the
   Earth Angel, to enter into the disharmony the earth
   is suffering and transform it from within. Ask
   Raphael in his Merlin guise to work closely with
   Sandalphon, and to bring the healing forces of his
   secret queen to bear upon the afflicted portion of
   the earth you are seeking to cleanse. Appoint the
   healing angels to stand guard over the vicinity until
   the healing begins to take effect. Hold all in the
   light of the star, and enquire of Archangel Michael
   once more, after the passing of a month, if your
   cleansing ritual may go ahead. If the answer is still
   negative, keep the healing angels in place via your
   specific instructions, and wait. Your inner direction
   as to how to proceed will make itself known at the
   right time.

Your intuition will guide you as to why Archangel Michael is advising against the cleansing ritual. When the time is right, follow the instructions given below.

The Cleansing Ritual

This is very simple. It has four stages, although it may not be necessary to implement them all.

Stage One

1 Imagine that you are holding a white rose bush, budding and ready to bloom. The white rose is the symbol of Archangel Michael. Call on him for protection as you enter the site of the disturbance you seek to heal. Surround yourself with light.

2 Ask the angels to guide you to the point of greatest pressure concerning the contamination.

3 Walk three times around it in a clockwise direction, and call down Archangel Sandalphon's blessing upon it, intoning the name with resonance.

4 Invoke the blessing of Raphael and his company of healing angels, followed by a request to Merlin and his secret queen to bless, heal, and to earth the angelic emanations into the pressure point. Chant the angelic names. Also call on the angels of purity.

5 Take your white rose tree, and plant it at that exact spot. Water it with ethereal water, and feed it with the starlight in your heart. Watch as it springs into the loveliest white blooms. Lovingly command the white rose tree to give forth its fragrance in full measure. Delight in this cloud of incense as it rises.

6 Summon the healing angels to assume stations of

protection and maintenance of the healing power until all is harmonious again. Give them this instruction clearly and directly.

7   Call down a blessing from Valoel, the great Angel of Peace. 'Under your white wings may this place be soothed into tranquillity, and receive your calm and stillness into its troubled breast. Amen.'

8   Thank the angels.

This little ceremony can be conducted when you are working alone, or with others when Archangel Michael has instructed you to work as a group. In the latter case, each member of the group will plant a white rose tree in the troubled area, as almost certainly there will be more than one pressure point within it. You can chant the angelic names to good effect when you work alone, but when you work as a group your chanting can become deeply musical and rhythmic, and will be very powerful.

This ritual can be enacted even when a trapped soul is present in the room or vicinity, because it can do no harm. Nevertheless, always ask for Archangel Michael's judgement of the situation before proceeding with any ceremony.

Stage Two

This simply involves waiting. Let one week or one month pass, whichever you feel is appropriate. If you are dealing with a trapped soul, you need only wait for three days. Return to the site, and test its energies, which may have healed by the enactment of the white rosebush ceremony alone. If the atmosphere is still stagnant, heavy or oppressive, follow the steps given above to ask Archangel Michael whether it is safe for

you to proceed to the third stage. If not, follow the
instructions as given above. If so, then you can proceed
as soon as it is convenient.

Stage Three (Group Work Only)

1 Elect a leader of your group, and let the rest of the
   group surround that person. From the centre, the
   leader will call on the blessing and protection of
   Archangel Michael. All members must see this great
   ring of white light descending. It forms a great cross
   of light within a circle of light. Go in imagination to
   the intersection of the cross, from which there blazes
   a single white star, pure and perfect. It is from this
   spiritual point that all must conduct the ceremony,
   meaning that in their spiritual awareness, that is
   where each member of the group must work from at
   all times. Never let go of your awareness of this
   blazing sacred centre, crossed and starred with holy
   light.

2 Proceed to the site of the problem. Stand together
   in a circle, and call on the Archangel Sandalphon,
   Archangel Raphael, and his company of healing
   angels, as before. Summon Merlin and the healing
   power of his secret queen to bless, heal, and to
   earth the angelic emanations into the site.

3 Chant all angelic names three times, or more if you
   feel a buildup of rhythm and power.

4 Call on the presence of the angel Tahariel, the
   Angel of Purity, to work her magic and give her
   blessing to your work and to the site.

5 Call on the angel Vywamus, the Angel of Cleansing,
   and give forth the invocation detailed in Chapter
   One.

6   Call on Zadkiel, Angel of the Violet Flame, to lend his mighty assistance. Invoke the Violet Flame ('I AM a being of violet fire. I AM the purity God desires'). Command the Violet Flame to cleanse and purge the vicinity.

7   Calling again on Archangel Michael, summon a whirling pillar of white light down from the heavens, from the third eye of the mighty Angel Michael. This white tornado, purer and brighter than any light on earth, stands spinning in the centre of your circle. Each member of the group must, with a huge release of willpower, command this tornado to move about the room, spinning with breathtaking rapidity as it sucks up and instantly transmutes all negative, contaminating energy into its twisting column of white flame. If there is any resistant energy, the tornado pulverizes it in a fraction of a second and scoops it up in its majestic whirlwind. Finally, it returns to the centre and becomes an angelic figure, sculpted of sanctified stillness and pure white fire, which spreads its arms and its wings about the affected area and about the group.

8   Command the healing angels to assume stations around the affected area, to conserve, maintain and direct the healing, cleansing forces until they have taken full effect.

9   Call down the blessing of Tahariel once again.

10 Thank the angels.

Stage Four

This is a repetition of Stage One, to be put into practice one week or one month after Stage Three.

The meditation poem that follows, concerning the mystic rose in our heart-centre, has been found useful by some as an inner focus prior to planting the white rose bushes of purification.

PEACE IS WITHIN

Find the point of peace within.

It dwells not in the mind,

Not in the turbulent emotional body,

But deep in the heart, like a tranquil jewel.

Give up the haughty claims of the mind,

Give up the anxiety-spell of the emotional body:

Go straight to the heart.

Like a babe enfolded in the embrace of its
mother,

Peace will hold you in everlasting arms;

It is a rose softly lit with the light of eternity.

Within its temple you receive true Selfhood.

Your in-breath partakes of its holy essence.

You breathe out its fragrance to heal the world.

Grounding Techniques

An essential for all healing work, and for our lives generally, is to learn to ground ourselves. Our tendency as human beings is to float off to some degree in our astral vehicle, and to semi-detach from our bodies. This does us no favours, because our destination, if we do float off, is an unreal state between the vital inner worlds of meditation and the fundamental physical world of earth. We truly inhabit neither when we are in this floating state, and we cannot ingest nourishment from either one. We are in a vacuum between earth and heaven.

To correct this state, we need to ground ourselves daily, and even more often if we ever feel particularly dreamy and detached. Some techniques are outlined below.

- A popular method is to imagine strong, fibrous, healthy roots growing from the soles of your feet and anchoring themselves deep into the essence of Mother Earth.

- Another way is to hold a grounding crystal (previously cleansed – just hold it under the flow of the cold tap for a second or two) such as bloodstone or smoky quartz in your left hand for a few moments until you feel steadied and centred.

- A third way is to affirm on the in-breath, aloud and whilst holding your right thumb and forefinger together, 'I am', and on the out-breath, 'present'. Do this three times.

- If you experience days when your energies feel severely unsettled, a little time spent in gardening (especially digging) or walking in nature will help you. You can always ask the earth angels to stabilize and earth such chaotic energies.

Cleansing the Aura

Many beautifully formulated sprays and perfumes are available nowadays which perform this function delightfully. However, they are expensive and not always easily accessible, so it is wise to have a stand-by. One tried and tested method is simply to rub the hands together briskly, as though you were seeking to create fire (which, of course, at the subtle level of life, you are). Smooth this subtle fire around the space at the top of your head and shoulders, vigorously chafe your hands together again, and continue down your auric field (the space around your body), pausing three or four times to renew the celestial fire in your palms before resuming your task. To treat the auric field that links with your back, simply stroke the space connecting to your neck and shoulders in a downward motion and see the spiritual fire streaking down your back. Lift the soles of your feet and pass your palms under them. You will note that we use the special, magical chakras in our hands to perform this method of aura cleansing; those chakras connected to our Vivaxis of which we will have so much to learn as the century unfolds.

Other methods of aura cleansing are the petition to Vwyamus, the Violet Flame ritual (*see* Chapter One) and the ceremony entitled 'the Dance of the Two Dragons' in Chapter Four. This petition, and the two ceremonies, are well worth using as often as we can. They will give us inestimable help in our development as angel healers, especially as so much of the angels' work on earth is concerned with the huge task of purification.

The Angel Altar

We need to create an altar, a magnetic point on which the angels are able to focus. The angels themselves have asked us to build and dedicate these 'magnetized centres'. Choose a corner of a room dedicated exclusively to the angels.

Clear this space with the techniques given above, and summon angels of protection to stand in the east, west, north and south. Lovingly command them to remain in place, protecting and energizing your altar at all times. Ask them to create and maintain a force around this corner of the room which will take the form of translucent walls. Cleanse your angel shrine (which is what your dedicated corner has now become), keeping it spotless and pristine as an angel would clean it: as a form of benediction and ritual, as a holy rite. Keep everyday thoughts, moods and activities away from the altar. Have on it:

- a white cloth
- perfumed oil, particularly rose and lavender, or a fragrance of your choice
- candles, white and gold
- holy water in a crystal bowl, which will be spring or mineral water that you have previously blessed by holding the filled bowl to your heart-centre and shining the symbol of the cross of light contained in the circle of light into the depths of the water; this has to be performed with love, and with reverence for the element of water
- fragrant flowers
- a symbol or a figure of the spiritual spheres which inspires you – perhaps from your religion, such as the Virgin and Child, a figure of the Goddess, one of the saints, a great teacher or prophet, one of the ascended masters, or one of the great humanitarian heroes (Martin Luther King, Mahatma Ghandi, Mother Teresa, etc.)
- a single object of great beauty, mentally associated with the angels and with nature
- an angel picture, or a symbol or design that reflects the angelic nature
- a golden dragon or serpent, which you will place towards the west of the altar (you can buy a dragon ornament and paint it gold, or create a makeshift serpent from golden thread or foil)
- dedicated and cleansed crystals (see Chapter Eight

on crystal healing webs to learn how to do this),
especially a clear quartz point and pieces of rose
quartz; you may like to use angel designated stones
such as celestite and angelite.

Place the altar to the east, and attend with angel invocations
once in the morning and once in the evening. If these are
intoned at sunrise and sunset, the healing power channelled by
your magnetized altar will be greatly increased. No doubt it will
not often be possible to enact the whole ceremony. Nevertheless,
if you aim for the fulfilment of this objective just once every
month, or even every three months, it will give a tremendous
boost to the magnetism of your altar. The magnetizing process
will take place as you attend to your altar and use it day by day.

The following ritual comprises an old ceremony you might
like to use.

MORNING INVOCATION

Hail, great Raphael!

Greetings, angels of the Healing Art!

Pour forth your healing life

Into… [name of person].

Let every cell be charged anew

With vital force.

To every nerve give peace and strength.

Let tortured sense be soothed.

May the rising tide of life

Set every limb aglow,

As, by your healing power,

Both soul and body are restored.

Leave here an angel watcher

To comfort and protect.

Hail, great Raphael!

Greetings, angels of the Healing Art!

Come to our aid,

And share with us the labours of this earth

That the indwelling God might be set free in
humankind.

AMEN

The officiant should speak the words with joy, and use all the
imagination, will, and the summoning power of the voice in
calling on the angels, whilst simultaneously raising the bowl of
flowers above the head and following them with the eyes.

EVENING PRAYER

May blessings from above

Flow forth and beautify the human love

Which we in gratitude pour forth

To you, our angel helpers of this day.

At the closing of this day

Be with…[name of person]

And draw your mantle of comfort,

Of protection and love

And gentle guidance from the higher planes

Around all those who suffer,

All those who are alone or afraid.

AMEN

Let the officiant hold up the bowl of flowers, offering their sweetness and their beauty to the angels, and pouring through them deep love and gratitude from the heart towards the angel hosts. Then give thanks in silence.

Adapted from *The Coming of the Angels*,
Geoffrey Hodson

The underlying law of creation is that the lesser must invoke the greater, reflected by the scientific rule that power always flows from the stronger to the weaker domain. This law is brought into operation by the force of prayer and invocation. Without them, we cannot work with the angels. It is vital to use prayers and invocations to initiate and accompany our angel communion.

When you use your altar for healing rituals, begin by lighting the white and the gold candles and greeting the angels of the cardinal points by bowing your head to each.

Say:

'My Guardian Angel, please link me to Archangel Raphael and his-her host of Healing Angels.'

Then intone three times, with intent, so that the angels can make a channel from your willpower to act on your behalf:

'May this altar be consecrated by the angelic host.'

Then say clearly, with your mind focused sharply on the words and what they mean:

'Archangel Raphael, I invite you into this sacred space. May it be a channel and a focus for you and your healing brethren to bring angelic healing forces to all who are present, or who are named, herein. I offer my thanks from a true heart overflowing with love for the angels and with joy in their presence.

Amen.'

Repeat the above invocation, this time to the Angels of the Rays.

Sprinkle the holy water in a circle, and create the sign of the cross within it, using your cleansed, blessed and dedicated clear quartz point. Do this three times.

Then anoint the centre of the imaginary cross with the perfumed oil, and place a flower there.

Bow to Raphael and all invoked angels, and move away from the altar without turning your back.

An angel invocation must be said in the morning, and a prayer of thanksgiving at night (*see* above). Adapt shorter ones of your own, to say when time is scarce.

You will note that you are expected to express joy, thankfulness and love during these rites. We cannot always feel these profound, abundant emotions, especially on demand! The trick is to *act* as if we are feeling them. When we act with true intent rather than in order to deceive, the act itself forms a channel through which higher beings can nourish us with the genuine essence of what we are expressing. This is the great difference between dramatic art and hypocrisy, and the secret as to why great actors can move us so deeply.

Robes

It is better if you conduct your angel ceremonies whilst barefoot, but you may also like to wear a robe. This is ideal, as robes can be ritually blessed and consecrated. If you find it too demanding a task to change in and out of robes twice a day, you might like to wear them only during your healing ceremonies. Never be put off your development as an angel healer by what might seem to be an inordinate tax on your time and energy. It is much better to cut, adapt and shorten all procedures as you need to.

Let your robe be simple and light, preferably white with a gold motif, which should be a symbol with which you resonate. Try to ensure that it is made from natural fibres, or as nearly natural as possible. Man-made fibres definitely inhibit spiritual work. If you have a favourite colour and you feel that your angel healing robe should reflect this hue, then choose a delicate, pastel shade. There should be no brashness, glare or opaque depth in the colour you choose. Nevertheless, white, with a touch of gold, is generally the best choice concerning ceremonial robes involving work with angels. Healers from the angelic realms will reflect colours onto you and your altar so that they may be given to your patients or healing projects, and the white light radiating from your heart and your robe forms the best receptacle for this procedure.

Wash your robe after every major healing ceremony (if these have to continue daily for a time, wash them every few days). Bless and consecrate your robe after washing by taking it to your altar and calling down a blessing from Archangel Raphael and Christ-Brigid, the Great Golden Healer of the Sun. (If you object to Christian terminology, you might like to use the term 'the Spirit and the Bride'.)

Afterwards, ask the angels to sanctify your robes in the same way as you asked them to sanctify your altar:

'May this robe be consecrated by the angelic host.
I dedicate its use to Archangel Raphael and his-
her Company of Healing Angels.'

Intone these words three times.

The Healing Temple

When we offer healing to ourselves or to others, whether they
are human or animal friends (or indeed strangers), a plant or a
tree, a garden or a place in nature, a house, a hospital, some
other building or gathering place, a village, a town, a city, a
country or even the planet, we are taken up by the angels with
our patient into a healing sanctuary in the angelic realms. It may
seem rather strange to think of some of the items listed as being
lifted into a healing temple, but the temple is deeply magical,
with the fairy quality of appropriate expansion and contraction,
so all are admitted!

It is helpful to form an idea of this temple. It is often perceived as a round white dome, with its roof open to the golden
sun. Around this sun are many stars, but we do not need the
darkness to see them, as we do on earth. The sun is set in a
perfect blue sky, a sweet and heavenly blue that flows down from
the skies as a calming, healing essence. The temple is filled with
niches or cells, as in a beehive, although each is set under a
window overlooking a wondrous garden of the spirit, beyond
which are white-capped mountains and springtime green forests.
The mountaintops are not covered in snow, but in angelic whiteness, unearthly, soft, and yet brighter than any light on earth.
Each one is a place of sanctuary, where sanctified minds can
retire and rest in visions of the supernal worlds.

Within the cells in the temple are soft, firm couches, where
the patient is gently laid by the attendant angels. The sun begins
to reflect most glorious and heavenly rainbow colours down

through the dome of the temple, which is roofed in a substance clear as clearest glass, but which bears the essence of water – a spiritual water that does not fall or make wet. Its translucency is a marvel to see.

The colours that cascade down from it are the most beautiful hues conceivable. Many of them are not visible on earth. To get a feeble idea of this wonder, fill a clear-glass bowl with water, and put into it crystals of many different colours, particularly delicately coloured ones. Their beauty under clear water will particularly delight you. (You may like to place such a bowl of crystals in water on your altar, to remind you of the healing temple.) The patients enter a healing sleep, in which they are lifted into even higher dimensions (if you look out of the window of one of the little healing shrines, you might see their souls in rapture on the mountaintops!). Meanwhile, they absorb the exquisite colours, as lovely as the angels themselves, deep into their chakras and their subtle bodies (each subtle body is attached to a chakra). When the healing treatment is over, the patients are gently withdrawn from the temple and escorted back into their physical bodies on earth.

Think often of the healing temple in the angelic worlds, and you will gain access to it for yourself and your patients all the more readily and easily.

Unfurling our Wings

We have angelic wings that we can unfurl and wrap around ourselves, creating a pillar of light in which we are completely protected. Positive emanations can come to us in our pillar of light, and we can give forth the radiance of our spirit from within its shelter, but negative, harmful thought-forms and vibrations are repelled.

It is easy to learn how to unfurl our wings. After the following exercise has been completed, it can be done anywhere, in an instant. Take care to make use of the shielding quality of your wings. As angel healers, we need to make sure that our chakras and auric space are kept as pure as possible, and that random attacks from thought-elementals and other pollutants don't drain our energy so that we are unable to carry out our work with the angels.

Our wings run from the base of our brain to the base of our spine, but when fully opened and extended, they can enclose our entire body from our earth chakra below our feet to our star chakra above our crown (these are reflections of the base and crown chakras).

> **Ground yourself (see above for grounding methods).**
>
> **Connect your heart, throat and crown chakras with a spiritual line of light.**
>
> **Breathe the light down your spine.**
>
> **Sense your spine alight and brilliant like a golden rod, all aglow with an influx of divine light.**
>
> **All the way down your spine, little golden seed-pods of light are bursting into wing-fibres.**
>
> **Let them extend to each side.**
>
> **See them growing into huge, full-length wings.**
>
> **Waft them, and feel their dimensions.**
>
> **Now wrap them right around yourself so that you are in a pillar of light.**

Once you have introduced yourself to the concept of your wings by working through this exercise, there is no need to go through each step when you wish to surround yourself with your pillar of light. Just command your wings to encircle you.

The Angelic Colour Spectrum

As healers working with the angels, either for ourselves or others, we need to know how to command and direct the colour rays – through *hands* and *thought*. The angelic colour-rays are very subtle, varied and beautiful, and have to be summoned from the imagination. It is in this area that the rainbow chalice (the heart receiving and transmitting the angelic colours) comes into play.

We have already encountered the rainbow chalice in a former exercise. For our angel healing programme, we need to deepen our awareness of it, and the colours that play within it and pour forth in abundance from it. Although when we are working with the angels, we need to learn how to convey the colour rays through our hands – and our thought, which we must train to be as clear and pure in its focus as crystal – we will always summon them from the rainbow chalice in the heart.

The seven rays of colour within the white light are headed by seven great planetary angels, who each command countless angelic hosts. The healing angels bear the colour to us that we select for our healing purpose, coming to us from the angelic host and the angelic head of that ray. We receive the ray into our heart from the six-pointed star, which shines above us as well as in our hearts. The great star, shining white at first, fills with the beautiful translucent colour of the ray we summon and pours it into our heart, into our rainbow chalice, where the colours rise and play and sparkle like jewelled fountains flashing in an urn wrought of bright mirrors and clear crystal. From there, our thought, our imagination, our breath and our hands direct it to the one who suffers, whether present or absent.

Let us look at the colours and gain a deeper insight into their meaning.

Blue

Blue is the colour of peace and serenity. It enfolds, as the blue sky endomes the world. It stills violence and agitation. Its healing flow is cool and calming. It returns us to stillness and silence. It denotes air, and puts us in mind of great airy spaces, clear, unobstructed, free of the strife and turmoil of our earthly concerns. Blue denotes air.

The quietude of blue can be brought to us on our breath, and circulate our system like a blessing from the Angel of Peace. It can be given to the solar plexus to calm emotional disturbance and strain, to soothe the jangling that often occurs in that centre and to help it to produce the right note once again. It can be given to the throat to ease nervousness, stress and tension. It can be given to the heart to clear from its well-shaft the accumulation of worry and fretfulness which prevent us from properly contacting our heart-centre. It can be given to the spine to wash and restore to its wisdom the whole chakra system. It can be given locally to soothe pain.

Blue is associated with wisdom, with teaching, and with high spiritual values. The Sapphire Tablet was said to be the source of Solomon's renowned wisdom, and the root of Hebrew mysticism as expressed in the teaching of the cabala.

Shades vary from holy or Madonna blue, the blue of summer skies to gentle, light blue – a delightful pastel shade sometimes seen in the sky at dawn on bright mornings when the land is covered in snow or hoar frost.

Green

Green is the colour of empathy, harmony, surrender, particularly the power of wilful surrender, which is immense. It denotes water. It is the heart-point of the rainbow, and the secret of the Earth, for green is her colour. The secret is that the Earth Being herself belonged to the domain of the Spirits of Water before she ensouled our planet, and that we, as human beings on earth, are all Children of Water.

In the vision of the prophet Ezekiel, when the angels showed him the four cardinal points, which denote the elements as well as the directions, he saw a man in the west, the place of water, although an ox, an eagle and a lion were placed at the heads of the other cardinal points.

Green is our special vibration. The fairies call the dimension in which we live, 'the Green World'. Green links us to nature. It is the colour of purification and compassion.

It can be given to clear congestion due to stress and tenseness, rigidity, brittle mind-sets, or to oversensitivity (bronchitis and asthma are often caused by these factors). It can be given to the spine, the throat and the solar plexus, and also locally, to cleanse and disperse inflammation.

It is the ray of harmony. The teacher White Eagle calls it 'an expression in form of higher things'.

The greatest wisdom – all that is known on earth and shall ever be known – was inscribed on the Emerald Tablet by Tiamat, the mysterious Dragon Queen, 'she who bore them all'. Tiamat was the great mother of all beings upon the earth, and she gave her precious Emerald Tablet into the safekeeping of the Annunaki, the god-people whom she summoned to earth at the beginning of time to initiate earth's humanity. It became known as 'the Emerald Tablet of the Annunaki', but was lost to the earth.

We dispense the holy green ray in shades of springtime green, sunlit green and shining emerald green.

Gold & Sunlight

These are classed together, although gold is the more vital of the two. Imagine angelic gold of a spiritually molten brilliance, exquisitely rich in quality. It can be sent to the spine and the head-centres, and to local areas where severe and stubborn conditions have taken hold.

It signifies spiritual wisdom and divine intelligence, and gives confidence in the loving care of the Great Spirit. Being touched with gold connects us with the angels so that we are lifted up into angelic fields of light and angelic golden joy. Such an out-pouring of angelic gold brings happiness, a lightening of the human situation, the instigation of hope.

It sweetens harsh critical thought and very fixed opinions and mindsets, and breathes a shimmer of gold into mourning, depressed, grief-stricken hearts, so that they begin to see the sun again.

Sunlight bears the same quality, but it is filtered through a softer medium. Where gold is vital, dynamic, potent, and vibrantly applied, sunlight kisses, caresses, and enfolds. Both rays can be applied to the adrenals (sited in the back, just above the kidneys) with good effect, as worry, fear, frustration and depression work through them and affect the kidneys.

Gold denotes fire, of course, solar gold from the Source of All, the inconceivable fire of the Godhead.

Orange & Red-Orange

These are the colours of vitality and foster the renewal of vigour. They bring fresh life force to the whole being, and can be given as a stimulating tonic. They are very enlivening and good for depletion on all levels.

They combine red and yellow: respectively, the life force of the body and the life force of the mind. It is interesting to note that farmers and organizers carry this colour in their auric field, especially organizers dealing in the field of nutrition. We can see how farming and food organization require both the earth or body forces and the forces of the mind, and how they combine to create nourishment for the human vessel. This mental and physical food is available to us in its ethereal essence from the orange and red-orange ray.

Can we imagine orange healing angels? They are like bright

tongues of orange flame, offering us an orange from their hands! Taste the keen zest of the orange,' they say. 'It bears our essence and our gift of mental and physical vigour.'

When the sun goes down, it sinks from its yellow height (higher mental and spiritual) into the bowels of the earth (the red earth force), and becomes like an orange ball This is the great task of the angels of the orange ray – to bring the exalted dynamic of mind – the mind in the heart, whose source is Love – down into the physical structure, so that it might throw off its rigid lifelessness and become imbued with spiritual vitality.

Carnelian and orange calcite resonate with this task. These crystals work with the angels of the orange ray, acting as receptacles, transmitters and transformers to aid the programme of this celestial endeavour.

The angels of the orange ray are angels of love, and indeed Love itself is the vibration of this ray. It denotes fire – the fire of the heart, holding the balance between earth and heaven. It can be given to the spleen as a wonderful overall energizer, a fillip for those who are weary and depleted and who may suffer from a run-down immune system. The spleen is located to the left of the back, slightly above the waist.

Amethyst

Amethyst is the colour ray that restores the soul. It brings acceptance and humility, inner strength and freedom from the enslavement of addictions. It gives us strength to endure difficult life situations, not in dreary resignation but in quiet faith that release will come when the moment is right.

It awakens hardened and closed hearts to new life and brings into springing vivacity from their fresh stirrings a delicate rainbow of hope and divine possibility.

This ray is given to the heart-centre to impart its sustenance and blessing.

Violet

This is a more intense and potent form of amethyst, and of course we know that the violet ray brings with it the priceless benediction of the Violet Flame Ritual (*see* Chapter One). Archangel Zadkiel is one of the guardians of this ray, and is working in close partnership with Archangel Raphael to bring healing, purification and renewal to humanity at this time.

The violet ray bears within its essence an immense potency of spiritual power and command, which we might guess from its identity as the Ceremonial Ray – the ray of Beauty. True beauty – beauty of thought, beauty of motive, beauty of content, purpose and language, beauty of the heart and soul which employs it – is the magic that activates the mystical violet ray. Selfish and objectionable forms of ceremony will reap the whirlwind.

The colour violet is associated with this supernal power of summoning the universal spirit of beauty, an all-pervading aspect of the Divine.

It cleanses, reintegrates, and liberates. It especially stimulates the heart and lungs, blessing them with purification and recuperative power.

We use the violet ray with care and discretion, because its healing power can be too purging. It is given to the heart-centre and the throat.

White Light

White light is the Christ light, which we shine from our hearts on those who suffer and seek our help. It is emitted from the star in the heart.

It can be used to tenderly enfold a patient, or, where powerful protection is needed, to blaze around them in the form of a cross contained in a circle.

We use the breath, and loving intention, to send this light to its mark.

Pearl

Pearl is the colour of the Christ Light which also carries a definite mother vibration. It is the love of Goddess, the Great Mother.

It gives stability and high aspiration, like a keen, sweet summoning of the soul by the noble ones of the pearlescent worlds, known to some as advanced fairy beings of great spiritual stature. It carries with it the magic touch of the Holy Spirit, light as a breath.

Its mysterious sheen is the soft, muted light of the wonders of the soul, yet to be unfolded.

We use pearl when the mother essence needs to be called upon to nurture the child within.

Rose

This is also the colour of divine mother-love, the gentle love which unites all humanity. We are familiar with the symbol of the rose, of course, and how it dwells in our deepest heart. We release the fragrance of the rose as a healing balm to those who have been hurt, abused, heartbroken. We gently enfold them in the rose ray, and usher them into the temple of the rose in the higher worlds.

When we need to call on the Sacred Feminine in our practice, we summon the soft rose light, glowing as if from an enchanted dimension where the angels move in hallows that are the dimensions of a rose that is the essence of loveliness, matter perfected and transmuted into the spirit of perfection itself. Such is the magic of the rose.

It is used to gently ease away blockages, and wherever there has been deprivation of love, especially in cases where patients have failed to love themselves. It is given particularly to the heart.

Silver & Flame

These are drastic and formidable cleansers. Silver projects the power and spiritual magnetism of the spiritual worlds into the lower earth-planes, whilst flame burns away dross and lights a pathway into the higher realms.

Both of these manifestations of colour appear in legend and folklore as fairy swords of terrible potency whom only the pure of heart could wield safely, without fear of the enchanted blades turning on their possessor.

Using the silver and flame rays in our healing work is perhaps not quite so dramatically dangerous, but nevertheless there is a wise teaching to be absorbed from the tales!

We implement them in cases of obsession and derangement, wherever unhealthy psychic conditions prevail. See a bright silver light or a flaming sword gently but briskly cutting away the etheric threads that link the patient with the undesirable condition. Imagine angelic hands over yours as you perform this healing rite, to prevent you from overdoing it! The safest way to use the sword is to carry out the procedure relating to the sword of Archangel Michael (*see* Chapter One).

Magenta

Magenta is the colour of the grand highway between heaven and earth, which unites the two.

The colour itself – deep rose, with a touch of violet – combines the first ray with the seventh ray of the seven great rays of creation. It is used to comfort and to restore balance, to stabilize and to steady a shattered or misaligned patient.

It links the organizing ability of the earth forces with the highest spiritual aspirations. It is worth bearing this quality in mind when seeking to help patients (you may encounter those who need to ground their dream of fulfilment, whatever that may be, in their practical existence, for instance).

Now that you have added the tools described above to your healer's treasury, and have contemplated the angelic colour spectrum and the mystery and beauty of the rainbow chalice, it is a good idea to have a practice run with it!

> Sit quietly, contemplating the star in the heart. Let your breathing be conducted through the peacefully shining star, so that your being fills with light on the in-breath, and gives forth light on the out-breath.
>
> Become aware of the mystic rose in your heart-of-hearts.
>
> The rose is opening out and giving forth a clear light until it becomes as crystal. It has assumed the shape of an exquisite chalice, flashing mirror-bright and clear as the purest glass. Around its rim are inlaid rings of diamonds and pearls.
>
> The star is now shining above your head. It pulsates with perfect light.
>
> Now the light is taking on the form of a rainbow. Its colours are delicate and jewel-bright, like spiritual mysteries. You are aware of angelic presences behind each ray. The awareness of them enters your heart like a cadence of joy.
>
> The colours begin to flow into the rainbow chalice. Soon they are dancing and playing in its sparkling depths, rising and spilling over the sides of the chalice in abundance, like enchanted fountains. The chalice mirrors and magnifies the magical colours, so that they gyrate and swirl around it like great dancing spirits performing rites of spiritual ecstasy around the ring of light in your heart.
>
> Choose one of these dream-bright colours, and summon it into the chakras in the centre of your

hands. Calmly breathe it into your waiting hands.

See it flow from the chalice in your heart into the still
pools of heavenly light that are the chakras in your
hands. There, the colour takes on the quality that the
angels breathe through it for your own or another's
healing: either gentle, virile, muted, star-bright, evanes-
cent with glittering motes of revelling energy, or calm
and tranquil as the first tender stars of a radiant
summer dusk. The hue changes with the mood and the
healing reverie of the angelic consciousness within the
vital heart of the colour.

Imagine conveying the colour to your patient, perhaps
to the spine or head area. Let this be an act of
profound self-giving, so that your heart-centre glows
even more brightly. Use the healing, blessing power in
your hands.

Let the colour pour into the centre in your patient that
you have chosen. Feel your link with the angels as they
modify the treatment, increasing or lessening the flow,
making the colour tone brighter or gentler according
to the requirements of the patient.

Give thanks to the angels for their healing and communion.

Step lightly out of your meditation, and seal your
chakras.

We will now progress to a study of the chakras – the next vital
step in attaining the goal of healing with the angels.

CHAPTER SIX

THE CHAKRAS

The angels work with us via our chakras, and so it is vital to attain a clear understanding of these centres which connect our physical being with our spiritual being in the higher worlds. When a person is unaware of their chakra points and is entirely uninterested in responding to the delicate vibrations of the worlds of the spirit, the chakras become clogged and murky. The energy that passes through them is dull and heavy, and they slowly become less and less able to do their work of linking us to our higher consciousness. As this process continues, the physical body becomes coarser and more gross.

When we activate our chakras, on the other hand, our material bodies become more and more refined, until finally those who encounter us can sense and even see the aerial play of these delicate rainbows of light that spring in a fountain from each of our centres. Others can directly receive refreshment, peace and healing from them even when no formal healing ceremony or procedures are involved.

There are many chakras, but most systems of spiritual teaching perceive the human structure as encompassing seven main 'star gates' or physical-spiritual points of contact. I would like to suggest that we need to think of eight main centres at this time, for reasons discussed earlier (*see* Chapter One in particular). This does not displace the idea of a construction of seven, but rather introduces the concept of the seven-and-one, which we might think of as manifesting as Earth and the seven planets in astrology that influence her. There are more than seven planets in our solar system, of course, but these more recently discovered planets actually reflect the qualities of the first seven at a higher level – in other words, they start to create a higher harmonic.

This idea is demonstrated clearly by the sol-fa system of notation, in which each note of an octave is designated a name from beginning to end (doh, re, mi, fa, so, la, ti, doh). Here we see that the final 'doh' is part of the octave, but is also the first note of a following higher harmonic. Thus, we see that music is constructed on the seven-and-one principle, in that it consists of the seven tones of music but completes itself in each harmonic (equivalent to a plane or sphere of being) by harmonizing the first note of each octave with the first note of the next octave in the scale (the final 'doh' in each case; if you sing the eight notes of the octave the explanation will become clearer).

Here we have a perfect mirror image of our chakra system, the seven-and-one, or the seven main chakras plus our earth chakra, which combines and reflects all of them in the magenta-coloured chakra which is connected directly to the earth through the Vivaxis. This chakra expresses itself through our hands and feet, the four chakras of which combine to make the one unified earth chakra, so giving us the cuboid, four-square symbol of the Earth herself.

The Earth Chakra

This chakra is located in the middle of the hands and the feet, upon the palms and the soles. Its colour is warm rose-magenta. We see this beautiful colour in the natural glass created by volcanoes, the fiery energy centres of the earth.

Its animal is the serpent, the Wise One. The Nephilim, or the Wise Ones, were the Serpent People who came to this planet in the beginning to initiate and nurture earth's humanity. They were of such an exalted evolutionary vibration that they resonated with the highest of the angels. Jesus and Mary Magdalene were of these Serpent People, the most honoured among them.

Their sign was the sign of these Wise Ones, the symbol of two fishes swimming in opposite directions, actually the sign of the serpent, associated with the caduceus and also with Pisces, emblem of the deeps of spiritual consciousness.

The energy flow to the earth chakra was obstructed before the coming of the Christ couple. The piercing of Jesus's hands and feet on his cross of sacrifice symbolize their gift to us of the restored flow of these energies, made complete by Mary's bringing forth of the essence which we lost when we lost the Grail. This essence was of the highest of the high within those deeps of spiritual consciousness, and had been given to Earth and her peoples in the beginning, in the days of Eden, but then brutally repulsed and driven out by the self-will of humanity itself. We will see, after the Grail has been recovered, that it was not so much a case of Adam and Eve (the leaders of humanity) who were driven out of paradise, but rather that human beings drove paradise out of themselves.

The Base Chakra

The first of the structure of seven chakras, the base chakra, is situated at the base of the spine, encompassing the little hollow there. It is linked with the planet Saturn. Its colour is a dramatic, rich, rubescent red. It is connected with the sense of smell, its element is earth, it is associated with Merlin and the Crone (the wise old man and the wise old woman), and its challenges are Fear and Darkness. We have to overcome our dark sleep in matter, and our fear of the spirit, at this level. We have to break out of our stupor, our unawareness.

The elephant is the sacred animal of this chakra. The elephant 'never forgets', just as we cannot afford to slip back into sleep and forget that we are spirit. We need the qualities of the elephant to master our lessons of this level: strength, wisdom, endurance and longevity of purpose.

The Sacral Chakra

The sacral chakra is located a little below the navel. It is linked with the planet Jupiter. Its colour is a glorious orange, shot through with brilliant crimson. It is connected with the sense of taste, its element is water, and it is associated with the gods and goddesses of humour, expansion, benevolence and exploration.

As well as its link with the sexual organs, this chakra encompasses the spleen, a very important organ which, at the subtle level of our being, is a transformer for the forces of wrath. This elemental force must be transmuted into love manifesting as peace. The roaring, fire-belching lower dragon must be resolved into peace, transformed into the love and wisdom of the Pendragon, who breathes forth the fire of the spirit, harming none and blessing all. This chakra might be called the centre of the feminine desire nature.

The animal of the sacral chakra is the alligator, which can manifest as the powerful and dangerous predator of the waters, lurking in their depths in wait for a chance to devour and destroy (just as wrath rises up and wreaks its havoc), or as the sacred dragon of peace and wisdom (the Pendragon).

The dragon is sign and symbol of Tiamat, the great Dragon Queen, who brings the great currents of life to humanity and to all the physical realm in their universal wave-form pulses (a manifestation of her sacred wavesque shape), and who is merciful, wise and all-encompassing in her love.

The Solar Plexus Chakra

The solar plexus chakra is located above the navel in the centre of the solar plexus.

It is linked with the planet Mars. Its colour ranges from green to golden green to warm, rich gold. It is associated with the sense of sight, its element is air, and it is associated with the gods and goddesses of courage, victory, willpower and achievement; those divinities who bless the questing soul and the pioneer.

The solar plexus chakra and the sacral chakra are connected by a large network of nerves, and both are associated with the two aspects, lunar and solar, of our desire body. The feminine, lunar sacral chakra reflects the masculine, solar third chakra, and this solar plexus centre tends to oxygenate the reflected lunar fires of the second chakra. These centres thus feed one another, creating chaos in our lives until we overcome their sway, upon which they metamorphose into peace, wisdom and love.

The sacred animal of the solar plexus chakra is the ram, the beast of sacrifice, for the lower fires must be sacrificed to the divine flame in the heart. When we do this by consciously choosing responses which are not centred in wrath and ego, the ram attains its golden fleece.

The Heart Chakra

The heart chakra is located in the centre of our chest. It is linked with the sun, the golden, perfected being which each of us is destined to become, the beloved Son-Daughter of Goddess-God, and its element is fire.

Its colour is a calm, clear, radiant gold merging into brilliant wine-red. It is connected with the sense of feeling and touch, its lesson is the ultimate expression of Divine Love – universal brotherhood – and its challenge is Lethal Jealousy (fear of death of the ego) and the fear of death itself.

The guardians of the temple of the heart are Saturn, Mercury and Venus. Saturn is the Alpha of the spine, Mercury is the Omega (in one guise, Merlin and Robin Hood, as we have discussed). At its midpoint, reflecting the heart-sun, is Venus, planet of love and harmony. Saturn, the stern old lawgiver, ensures that the heart obeys the Law of Love.

Mercury, at the top of the spine, is linked with the Archangel Raphael, as are both Merlin and Robin, and is the golden consciousness which has transcended the constricting chains of Saturn because his lessons have been learnt and the law is within his heart; it can no longer imprison him.

Venus is the point of balance between the two, the ascended soul who is yet alive in a physical body on earth. This is the ultimate goal of the heart – to spiritualize the planet itself, and exalt brotherhood to the point of celestial harmony.

The animal associated with the heart is the sphinx. This creature represents supreme consciousness rising from an animal body set four-square on the earth. In its most mystical aspect it signifies the fused being of the Spirit and the Bride – the heart-centre itself.

The Throat Chakra

The throat chakra is located in the hollow of the throat. It is linked with the planet Venus, the planet of love, harmony and beautiful creation. Its colour is fiery gold transforming into vivid lilac or ultraviolet.

It is connected with the sense of hearing and listening, its element is the white ether from which all form is birthed into being, and is also the space in which it is contained.

It is associated with Brigid or Bride (the Daughter) and Divine Mother, the Great Goddess herself. Its lesson is that of harmonious union, and its challenge is the power of the flesh, or enslavement to the body.

Venus brings us the blessing of Silence, the spiritual dimension of peace, whose magical point we find in the heart. When we enter into this Silence day by day, we can learn to overcome the challenges of the throat centre, so that the flesh no longer enslaves us, and we are at peace in our spiritual home as we walk the good earth.

The Brow Chakra

The brow chakra is known as the Third Eye, and it is located at the midpoint of the brow above the eyes. It is linked with the planet Mercury, the messenger, and with the sixth sense. It also receives the influence of the planet Uranus.

Its colour is a perfect rose hue, as the first blush of sunrise. It is known as 'the abode of joy', and it is a centre of command. Mercury's mission is to enlighten us through the brow chakra with sudden, sometimes shattering, illumination and revelation.

'Foolish wisdom' is the challenge of the sixth chakra – knowledge gained from earthliness but unenlightened by intuition and understanding and awareness of the spirit. Materialist science and medicine, technology that takes no account of ecology, are full of such 'foolish wisdom'.

The creature of the sixth chakra is the hawk, or the white eagle. From its great and noble height, far above earthliness, its eagle eye can spot every detail below on earth. It has not lost sight of earth, but it is aloft, in the heavens, riding the spiritual winds in freedom.

The Crown Chakras

There are two crown chakras. The first is in the middle of the brain, and takes the form of a full moon. From this full moon there grows the horn of the moon spirit-animal, the mythical unicorn. Our unicorn's horn is the second of this double crown chakra. It is located at the top of the forehead, at its midpoint. The crown with its diadem is a symbol of these two chakras, and illumines their form and purpose, which is to receive the divine illumination of the stars and the supernal glory which shines behind their manifestation, and to give forth the light of Christ Consciousness so that the individual can take his or her place among the radiant stars. The physical universe is a representation in matter of what we shall become – the starry celestial company creating the radiance of heaven.

Both of these chakras (the composite crown chakra) are associated with the moon. Influences from Neptune and Mercury also govern these centres.

Their colours are as a mystical rainbow, even more lovely than the natural phenomenon. Their lustre shines with every combination of colours that we know on earth, and scales of colours beyond these that admit more and more light until the rainbow itself is transfigured. They also manifest the Christ Light, the perfect white light, sometimes pearly, sometimes with a breath of brightest silver, and sometimes what I can only call a 'glad' light which pours gloriously forth as if it cascades from the Holy Grail.

The chakra at the midpoint of the temples – our unicorn's horn – is where we attain cosmic consciousness. The horn is like an omnipotent mast sweeping the starry fields of heaven. The chakra in the heart of the brain, which is a reflection of the 'nous' or the mind in the heart and is so strongly linked with the full moon, is also closely connected with hearing and listening. It is also a receiving and reflecting station which feeds the diadem whose central jewel is the point in the middle of the forehead between the temples, the flashing gem of divine wisdom.

This full-moon chakra is like a tranquil lake reflecting the light of the spiritual star which shines above the head. Whilst we are unable to activate our chakras and pass through the 'nous', or the doorway into Silence that resides in the heart, in full-moon consciousness, our being is like the moon we see from earth – a beautiful shining entity which is gradually eaten by the darkness of the earth, but which is always reborn out of the belly of the night.

When we attain our fully illumined state, however, this natural ebb and flow is overcome, and the moon of our being remains imperishably full, just as we are one with the imperishable stars (the spiritual light of the celestial bodies). It is then that the chakra

above our crown can be seen – our soul-star chakra – pouring forth
its effulgence in a starburst of rainbow colours, exquisitely radiant
yet delicate, subtle, almost pearlized.

The interplay of these fountains of energy produces jewel-
like fireworks over the top of the head. The other chakras take
up the colours and each one spins in its own permutation of
light, colour and sound, fabulous to behold. The centres communicate with the body, and they communicate with the stars,
by throwing out those magnificent radiations beyond the auric
field. We need to understand that the chakras within us do communicate with the stars, and receive very beautiful star energies
into themselves, with which they imbue our consciousness. It is
a communication with God, with the Divine Spirit pervading
the cosmos.

The challenge of the crown chakra is self-righteous materialism, which manifests when a very narrow and bigoted sense of
divinity is all that is allowed to develop, or when the ego
mistakes itself for divinity, and pronounces its judgements (often
only a reflection of its likes and dislikes and the restrictions of its
viewpoint) as if on divine authority. Both of these states choke
the motion of the chakras and cause their energies to stagnate.

The lesson of the crown chakra(s) is the attainment of
cosmic consciousness through the development – in the heart –
of love, wisdom and spiritual willpower (the will-to-good), which
activate the chakras. The two animals connected with the two
crown centres are (mid-brain) the dragon and (mid-forehead)
the unicorn.

We can see how essential it is for us as angel healers to keep our
chakras cleansed and energized. Illness always manifests as an
imbalance in these centres, which poisons the aura. We must be
able to receive high-frequency energy from the spiritual
starlight directly into our centres, or we will become ill ourselves when we try to help others. To do so, we have to keep
them clean and clear.

Cleansing & Energizing the Chakras

Constant aspiration to uphold spiritual values and awareness in our individual lives is the only true method of keeping our chakras untainted, of course, but there are methods we can use to purify them on a regular basis, either gently or vigorously, as stated in each case.

Archangel Zadkiel (Vigorous)

This mighty archangel is drawing very, very close to us at this special and spectacular time in human history. She-He is the Archangel of the Violet Flame. Sit in quietude, light a white or a violet candle, and ask Archangel Zadkiel to cleanse and balance your chakras with the Violet Flame.

Vwyamus (Vigorous)

A petition to Vwyamus (*see* Chapter One) to cleanse and balance our chakras is a powerful method of discharging subtle negative matter from our chakras.

The Sword of Michael (Vigorous)

This cleansing sword can be used to clear our chakras. See the blade as flashing bright silver, flame, or gold. See it cutting away all unwanted attachments and purging all stagnant energy. Then seal your chakras and your auric field with the opposite blue edge of Archangel Michael's sword. (The auric field extends around our body space to the extent of a hand's length from wrist to fingertips – often to a far greater depth, but this is the point at which we need to cleanse and seal it.)

Archangel Michael's Lustral Fire (Vigorous)

For an explanation of this lustral fire, *see* Chapter Four under the headings 'Archangel Michael's Purifying Fire' and 'The Dance of the Two Dragons'. This is a wonderful way to cleanse and invigorate the chakras.

Angel Invocation (Gentle)

Use this angel invocation to cleanse and balance your chakras:

> 'Angels Trsiel [Tri-si-el], Rampel and Dara,
> [*chant all names three times*]
>
> send your mighty purifying flow of clearest crystal
>   energy
>
> along my spine and throughout every chakra,
>
> so that it flows as a lustral river at floodtide
>
> of angelic intention.
>
>
> 'Angel Nahaliel [Na-ha-li-el],
>
> Bring the blessing of the rapid flow of running
>   streams
>
> into each and every chakra of my being.
>
> Let your dancing, diamond-bright energy
>
> circulate through my chakras continually,
>
> fostering the radiant flow of the spirit.
>
>
> 'Angel Anthriel,
>
> bring your gift of balance and harmony

to each and every one of my centres.

Stay on guard, holy one,

sustaining and maintaining these gifts of your virtue

until I cleanse and balance my chakras again.'

Crystal Cleansing (Vigorous — for extreme cases of contamination)

Using a clear crystal quartz point which you have cleansed, dedicated and programmed according to the instructions given in Chapter Seven, move it anticlockwise around each chakra, whilst pointing your left hand down to the ground. Use your right hand to make the anticlockwise movements.

Concentrate on seeing all the accumulated negative energy in each chakra dispersing and flowing through your left hand into the earth, who whirls it away and purifies it. Then, with your right hand, move the crystal point clockwise around each chakra, cupping your left hand to receive angelic light from the higher worlds. Finally, make the sign of the cross over each chakra, and touch the centre of the cross with the tip of the crystal point.

Rose Tree Cleansing (Gentle)

Sit quietly, and breathe through the heart until you have found the point of peace within. See the form of the mystic rose appearing there, like a miracle. Imagine your spine as a tree, with your chakras flowering from it as exquisite roses, each opening from the delicate bud. Let the fragrance of the rose in your innermost heart give itself forth from each rose, bringing it tenderly into full bloom.

Star Cleansing (Gentle)

Follow the method outlined above, but see the light of the star in your heart bringing each rosebud into a perfect flowering.

Kyanite Wand Cleansing (Gentle)

Cleanse a piece of kyanite wand, according to the instructions given in Chapter Seven, before you begin. Sit in peace, breathing through the star in the heart. Hold the piece of kyanite wand for a minute or so in your left hand, and then in your right for a similar length of time. Ask the angels to monitor and modify the chakra cleansing and balancing process that is underway.

Vivaxis Cleansing for the Hands & the Feet

Even though we may have cleansed our chakra system as a whole by choosing one or more of the methods outlined above, and applying them daily, or at least as often as we can, it is still worthwhile to take special care of the chakras in our hands and feet.

This is our earth chakra, the first-and-last chakra that combines the colours of the first and the last of the seven rays of creation which express themselves through the rainbow, and through the seven main chakras, even though the colours of the rays and the colours of the chakras differ to some degree.

Through the chakras in our feet (in the middle of each sole), we receive important forces from the Earth herself that we use in our angel healing ceremonies. Through the chakras in our hands, located at the centre of our palms, the earth forces and the angelic powers from the heavenly realms combine. Our arms link our hands with our heart-centre, and from this crucial chakra our lustrous rainbow chalice overflows into our hands, so that we, through their medium, convey the necessary angelic colours to our patients. We will receive hidden colours from our rainbow chalice as well, colours ascending in secret scales of light from worlds beyond all imagining. As the century progresses, we will find that our hands are directly involved in the energy we need to release, and the consciousness with which we need to connect, in order to achieve ascension. Zadkiel, the great Archangel of Ascension, waits to help us in every way with this magnificent process.

To ensure that the chakra points in our hands and feet which comprise our earth chakra are cleansed and revivified every day, carry out the second part of the exercise in Chapter One, entitled 'Locating the Vivaxis', as a separate procedure in addition to any of the above exercises you may choose to perform.

After completing the chakra cleansing and balancing method of your choice, always remember to seal each centre with the symbol of the bright silver cross contained in a circle of light.

Our chakra energies should take the form of glorious fountains springing up from the base of our spine through the heart, branching from there into three dancing and brimming spouts as they rise up through the head-centres. Each chakra should look like a liquid firework display of rainbow colour, whirling dance and heart-striking musical cadence. To help us achieve this goal, we can work through the following guided visualization as one of the means by which we seek to activate our chakras.

The Crystal Stairway

Begin to breathe peacefully, through the heart, until the door to the Silence opens and you are admitted therein.

You are standing upon the good earth, under an open sky, looking up at the blue heavens.

A crystal stairway of supernatural beauty winds in a spiral from the earth up into the celestial blue. Up and

down this wondrous stairway, angels of radiant loveliness and mystical presence come and go.

As you watch them in wonder, you see that there are
seven great steps which compose this magnificent
crystal stairway.

The stairway gleams sometimes as pure and translucent as a diamond, and sometimes with a bright
white purity as it reflects the brilliance of the angels.

You set your feet upon the first stair.

You see an angel of earth, calm and lovely, moving
towards you. She is red-cloaked and radiant, a marvel
to behold. You know that she is Sophia, Angel of
Wisdom.

She carries a ruby in her hand, and she places it in
your first chakra, at the base of your spine. The ruby
begins to glow a beautiful, clear red, like the heart of a
volcano seen through a spirit-bright mirror, and your
base chakra opens like a flower and begins to spin.
You see the crystal stair beneath your feet shine with
this wonderful, jewel-clear red, as beautiful as if it
flowed like a secret joy from enchanted lands.

As the crystal stair shines beneath you, bathe in the
colour; breathe it in.

'Your base chakra is cleansed and balanced, and
blessed by the angels. Stability is yours,' your companion tells you. You feel her great, rooted strength as she
withdraws.

You set your feet upon the second stair.

Another angel approaches, this time a sweet, peaceful
angel of water. She is Sachael, Graceful One of the
Waters.

She bears a magical, faceted gem of carnelian, glowing with the rapturous orange of a glorious summer sun sinking in a lake of red fire in the western skies. She places it in your sacral chakra, a little below your navel. The carnelian begins to pour all its vivid, vital orange and fiery red into your sacral chakra, so that this second centre opens like a flower and begins to spin. You see the crystal stair beneath your feet light up with this scintillating orange and crimson red.

As the crystal stair shines beneath you, bathe in the colours, breathe them in.

'Your sacral chakra is cleansed and balanced, and blessed by the angels. Peace and wisdom be with you,' says Sachael of the Waters as she withdraws, leaving you as if in a great calm ocean of peace and deep inner knowing.

You set your feet upon the third stair.

You see an angel of air approach you, with luminous flowing garments of softest blue streaming around her. She is Anael, Divine Protectress of Air, bearing a glittering jewel of yellow topaz, and a piece of precious jade with a pearly green translucence like a wave of the sea. She places both jewels in your solar plexus centre.

The topaz takes brilliant, flashing flame and the jade shimmers with the green dusky light of reflected suns as your solar plexus centre opens like a flower and begins to spin.

You see the crystal stair beneath your feet light up with this coruscating yellow, this green dim opalescent fire, softly auriferous.

As the crystal stair shines beneath you, bathe in the colours, breathe them in.

'Your solar plexus chakra is cleansed and balanced, and blessed by the angels. May you know the mystery of Love, both human and divine,' says the angel Anael, brilliant in her aerial beauty. She smiles, leaving you with her angelic blessing of love as she withdraws.

You set your feet upon the fourth stair.

This time, a glowing angel of fire, like a perfect, poised flame, draws near. She is the mighty Shekinah, Angel of Purest Everlasting Light. She carries an emerald of deep, luscious, light-filled green, secret in its depths with the wisdom of ancient sunlit forests and the life-bearing primal ocean. She places this precious jewel in her own heart-centre.

'What do you see?' she asks.

You see a Being of Light in her heart, greater than the universe. You know that this is the Dragon Queen, that we are all her Children of Light, and that each of us bears a drop of her essence in our deepest heart. It is the Divine Source.

You hear yourself say, 'I see the true centre.'

'You have answered well,' says the angel Shekinah. Her outline coruscates with holy fire; you see that she herself manifests the form of the Dragon Queen, Giver of Purest Everlasting Light, and that she, Shekinah, is its Shepherdess.

Shekinah holds forth a jewel in each hand, flashing in the centre of her palms. One is a citrine of calm, clear, radiant gold; the other is a light-filled garnet of a brilliant wine-red. She places both jewels in your heart-centre. In their radiant glow, your heart chakra opens like a flower and begins to spin. You see the crystal stair beneath your feet reflect these glorious colours and ray them out to the world as a wondrous red-gold.

As the crystal stair shines beneath you, bathe in the colour; breathe it in.

'Your heart chakra is cleansed and balanced, and blessed by the angels', says the majestic and gracious Shekinah. 'May the Love which unites all in brother-hood never grow dim within you.'

She leaves you as if in a miraculous cloak of all-enfolding brotherhood as she withdraws.

You set your feet upon the fifth stair.

An angel of the higher ethers floats tranquilly to your side, shining with a mystical purity. She is an angel of the hidden worlds, with a hidden name.

She places one jewel of fiery gold and another of pure deep amethyst in your throat chakra, at the hollow of your throat. Within the rays of that mystery of gold and violet, your throat chakra opens like a flower and begins to spin. You see the crystal stair beneath your feet flood with these colours and surround you as if with an aura.

As the crystal stair shines beneath you, bathe in the colours; breathe them in.

'Your throat chakra is cleansed and balanced, and blessed by the angels. May you know divine union,' says the Angel of the Hidden Name, leaving you with a feeling of great expanse as if you trod the unlimited fields of space: space fields filled with light, love, warmth and joy.

You place your feet upon the sixth stair.

A glittering sun angel, brilliant and lovely, moves to your side and reveals a jewel in her palm which shines as if it were a tiny stolen piece of the sublime spiritual worlds when they shine through the mystery of the dawn; a perfect sphere of most holy rose, fragrant and alive like the bloom itself.

The angel is Gazardiel, Angel of the Rising Sun, and she places the living wonder of the rose gem in your brow chakra, which opens like a flower and begins to spin, glowing with a deep rose hue of measureless beauty, which is reflected in the crystal stair beneath your feet.

As the crystal stair shines beneath you, bathe in the colour, breathe it in.

'Your brow chakra is cleansed and balanced, and blessed by the angels. Your third eye, the Abode of Joy, is open. May you be deeply blessed in your seeing,' says Gazardiel, Angel of the Morning; and as she withdraws you feel a surge of joy in your newly awakened state.

You place your feet upon the seventh stair.

A mighty angel of the sun, Brigid the White herself, approaches you on a white horse. Archangel Brigid shimmers pure white and glorious gold before you, beautiful as the sanctified mind of God.

She passes her hands over your head in blessing, and places a pearl of peerless beauty in the crown centre at the top of your head. She opens her other hand, and delivers a second pearl to the crown chakra in the middle of your forehead at the top, a pearl with a sparkling, fairylike sheen that, like Keats' dove of hope, fills the air with silver glitterings. Your crown chakras open like two perfect flowers and begin to spin, pouring forth a transcendent pearly light like a miracle, in which a silver lustre dances like a spirit. It illumines and floods the crystal stair under your feet.

As the crystal stair shines beneath you, bathe in the colour, breathe it in.

'Your crown centres are cleansed and balanced, and blessed by the angels,' Brigid the White, Angel of the Magnificence of the Sun, says to you. 'It is forever protected by me, and by my spiritual sword.'

Taking her sword of platinum gold from its diamond scabbard, she points upward.

'Behold, dear child of the pure and everlasting Light,' she says to you. 'You will see a vision, and experience a wonder. You are about to cross the rainbow bridge.'

Above her pointing sword shines the great star, all peace, all love, the Light of the World. It is the star that also shines within your own heart-centre.

Within its heart dwells Allea, the Great Angel of the Rainbow, and from the white light pouring from the star she creates the delicate hues of the rainbow; angel colours, many-splendoured with colours rising on scales of light into profundities of spiritual life where you cannot follow, although you can sense these transcendental colours and their sublime inner voyage at the very farthest reaches of your subtlest, intuitive vision. They are expressions of eternal Love.

Become aware now of your own individual star, shining in your heart-centre. Gently carry your breath to it, and breathe through it. It grows as you focus on it.

From the wondrous rose which blooms at the centre of the star in your heart, an arched bridge, seven-hued and seven-rayed, emerges. The arch of this miraculous rainbow reaches right into the centre of the great star above, and you see that Allea, the Angel of the Rainbow at the midpoint of that great star, is actually creating one half, and more than one half, of the arched bridge which leads from your star in the heart to her own heart-centre.

She holds out her hands to you, and you set your feet on the bridge.

You realize that your feet are winged, and you find yourself floating gently over the bridge into the vast star. And then, in great joy, you realize that the star in your heart and the great star are one, and you are safe and at peace in the arms of Allea.

She says to you, 'Ascend the crystal stairway, cross the rainbow bridge to the heavenly realms where the angels dwell to greet us whenever you wish, but remember always to make your heart your dwelling place.'

Bathe in the glory of the eternal star, and, when you are ready, gently return over the rainbow bridge, which has become the crystal stairway.

Descend to the violet stair,

down to the indigo stair,

down to the blue stair,

down to the green stair,

down to the yellow stair,

down to the orange stair,

down to the red stair

and back to earth, to the space you occupy and the here and now.

Seal your centres and, if you feel the need, root yourself into the earth by imagining strong, healthy, fibrous roots growing from the soles of your feet right down into the heart of Mother Earth.

CHAPTER SEVEN

THE HEALING POWER OF THE ANGELS

Up to this point we have discussed many important features of angel healing. It is time to learn the simple methodology involved in facilitating this potent source of therapy.

You have learned how to create and maintain an angel altar, and how to bless and consecrate your healing robes. You will have pondered on the miracle of the rainbow chalice and the angelic colour spectrum, whereby the angels use colour, some of it beyond our range of perception, to bring healing to the spine, the aura, and the chakras of those who suffer. You have learned how to cross the rainbow bridge into the angelic realms in order that you may activate your own chakras and allow them to communicate with the stars so that they receive vital spiritual energy, consciousness, and angelic emanations from the cosmos.

You have learnt the necessity of understanding the chakras, and of keeping them clean, balanced and energized, along with your aura and your healing environment, and how they all need to be protected. You have drawn close to your guardian angel, to Archangel Raphael and his company of healing angels, to Archangel Michael-Shekinah and to many other angels. You know the secret of the Spirit and the Bride, and how to call on this unified Being for healing, protection, guidance and blessing.

You have developed many healing tools: the star and the rose in the heart, the fragrance of the rose, the rose temple and the rose tree, an angel-inspired imagination, the rainbow chalice, the healing power of silence which is located through the 'nous', the mystical power of the breath, the sword of Michael, the power of the Violet Flame, the secret of the hands, the crucial need to utilize the act of prayer, invocation and meditation in your angelic contact, the magic of ceremony, and above all, you have learned how to withdraw to the centre of love, power and wisdom which is your heart.

Whether you decide to use your angel healing skills for yourself alone, or to convey them to afflicted members of your family and friends, or even to become a fully fledged angel therapist, you will need to absorb the following essential points.

Use Names

Always intone the name of your patient when you are invoking healing for them. Say it several times, as a chant, because you are summoning their soul. Employ a tone of authority and command (not dominance), because you need to stir and alert their soul. Their name carries a special vibration that directly links them with their higher soul. (Tennyson, a poet much more relevant to the present day than is suspected, always began work on his poems by calling his own name several times, in sonorous tones, to summon his higher soul).

This is especially necessary in absent healing, of course; and your healing practice should unfailingly include absent healing treatments for all patients, as well as face to face sessions. This might be said to be the most important part of their healing journey, although, of course, at the human level, it is very beneficial for patients to have the reassurance and the focus of healing treatments at which they are present. Even when this is so, it is still necessary to intone their name at the start of each session.

Materialism and Ego

Never allow money, or egotistical drive, to be your concern in giving angel healing. Maintain humility, and a deep respect for your patients, in every situation. If eventually you do become a paid angel-healer, never allow the business aspect of your work to be your main focus.

It is right that you should receive a reasonable standard of living for what you do; but let the desire to give pervade your heart and be your only inspiration, even whilst you quietly and efficiently deal with the economic aspect of your occupation.

Gain Experience

Practise on yourself first, before you move on to offering angel healing to friends, family, and those in need who hear that it is available! It is important that you feel happy, relaxed and familiar with all aspects of angel therapy, and that you have a degree of experience, before you convey them to others.

Understand Touch

The laying on of hands is not for everyone. Nevertheless, don't be discouraged concerning this aspect of the healing. Your hands secrete wonderful forces. If you feel unsure about this process, never force the issue within yourself.

You might like to start very simply and undemandingly by holding the hand of your patient for a few moments when giving healing, or just placing a hand on his or her forehead. Let the angels guide you as to whether you should offer the laying on of hands. Do only what feels comfortable for your patients and yourself. If a patient tenses when touched, try working with your hands just above the surface of their skin. You will in any case always use your hands in your absent healing rituals.

Use of Hands

If you do decide to use this method of healing, begin by placing both hands around the top of the head. Progress by descending to the forehead, and remain there for some moments. Tune in to the patient's third eye (the brow chakra), because it will have important information to relay to your intuition concerning the person's health, and the causes that lie behind the manifesting suffering and symptoms.

First of all, convey the loving light from the star in your heart to each chakra, and to the spine. As you do this, you will receive thought-messages from the angels concerning the colours and the appropriate chakras to which they ought to be conveyed. You may feel the need to rotate your hand lightly over each chakra. Always do this in a clockwise direction (moving from left to right).

Feel the colours coming from the angels into your rainbow chalice, and then flowing from there into your hands and into the patient. Always envisage calm, radiant, delicate colours, and let them gently, caressingly, enter each designated chakra. Prior to this treatment and to the arrival of your patient, of course, you will have washed your hands both physically and ritualistically, using one or both of the hand-washing ceremonies given in Chapter One.

You will also have called on Archangel Raphael and his company of healing angels, and on the angels of the rays, using the invocations given in Chapter Five, or invocations of your own. You will have prepared for your healing ceremony by cleansing yourself, your aura and your chakras, the room in which your angel altar resides, and by making a careful study of the information given in Chapters Five and Six concerning the chakras and the angelic colour spectrum in particular relation to the patient you are preparing to treat.

Understand the Patient's Need

When a patient applies to you for help, or when you wish to use angel therapy for yourself, gather as much information as possible about the kind of healing needed. This can be achieved by listening to the patient, or to your own symptoms, with the careful attention of the inner ear. Remember the centres which help us to listen with ears that hear: the throat, the brow and the crown centres, all activated from the heart, the seat of intuition (inner tuition).

The angels help us to build into ourselves those qualities that we lack, and which are creating the difficulty or illness that needs to be healed. For instance, worry and depression can be tackled by building faith, courage and joy into our nature. The angels help us to do this by teaching us to summon the specific angel we need (the Angel of Joy, the Angel of Faith, the Angel of Courage, etc.) and to absorb the energy or light-ray of the angel directly into our soul, which is achieved by attunement to the angelic worlds through meditation and star breathing (*see* Chapters One and Two) and by treating the appropriate chakra or chakras (*see* Chapter Five). Which angel do you or your patient need? What are the colours you need? Which chakras would benefit most from receiving the colours? There will be many clues to guide your deductions, but let the latter be made with the help of the angels. Listen to them as you formulate your judgements.

The Healing Process

You might address a healing situation in the following way: What is the real cause which lies at the root of the problem?

Is it anger, or resentment because of a sense of injustice?

You will need blue, to calm the anger; rose, to reassure and turn away wrath; amethyst, to open the heart and bring in a sense of the bigger picture, whereby our experiences in life sculpt and hone our soul, and bring to life its beautiful gifts. A touch of angelic gold, the essence of happiness, would surely help this patient to see their situation in a new light.

Blue and gold are given to the spine, so you would treat the spine by shining these rays upon it (they are given together).

Rose and amethyst are for the heart, so the rose-amethyst ray would come into operation here. Finally, you would hold the patient in the shining heart-light of the Spirit and the Bride.

Which angel would you call upon, as well as Raphael and her-his healing angels, upon whom we always call in healing situations?

Surely the Angel of Forgiveness is needed here, and also the Angel of Peace?

The Angel of Love would help this patient to feel loved again, because the apparent injustices of life make us feel victimized.

The Angel of Wisdom would assist the patient to see their situation in a clearer, more impersonal light.

And, as anger and resentment have taken root, you would do well to summon the Angel of Humility, who helps us to move away from the narrow stance of the ego, to bless this patient.

During your healing ceremony, all of these angels would be invoked for the sake of the patient, to bless and to heal. You would turn to your altar, and direct their beneficent influences through the flowers, through the crystals, through the candle flames, through the energy of the symbols and persons represented on the angel altar, so that the benediction of the angels invoked will be magnified and directed through the clearest possible focus.

You would then think of the angels of the seven rays. The rays of love and wisdom are required in this case.

You would thus call upon angels of the orange ray (a ray of love), and angels of the blue ray (a ray of wisdom) to select members of their order to stand by and remain with the patient until the healing was complete.

You would finish your healing ritual by educating the patient in a simple and kindly way – certainly not lecturing! – but rather teaching the patient how to sit and absorb the love of the angels, and to understand that they are an ever-available source of love and compassion for us constantly to draw upon;

also by explaining gently that we have to be prepared to let go of bad energy before we can be healed. The angels will help to enlighten you in your education of your patient.

Finally, you would offer your endeavours to Archangel Raphael and his circle of healing angels, and leave the matter in their hands. End with a dedication of thanks to the angels, and to Divine Spirit.

Preparation

Before your patient arrives and you begin your healing ceremony, stand before your altar and verbally invoke all the power available for the purpose of the healing work you are about to undertake. We identify the sources of power as:

1 The Godhead, and the God power within each one of us, which is inexhaustible and without limit. We connect with this divine source by withdrawing into the heart.

2 The power of the Logos of our system, whom we can directly contact through calling on Christ-Brigid, or the Spirit and the Bride. Again, we make the connection through our heart chakra.

3 The power of our religion and its founder, whether we belong to one of the established religions, or whether we express our spirituality as a love of nature (in which case, we might call on Mother Earth herself as our 'founder'). Geoffrey Hodson tells us that calling on our religion and its founder, if our religion is a living reality in our lives, will unfailingly produce a descent of power, and that there is a reservoir of power behind every religion that works for the upliftment of humanity. We tune into the religion's 'higher self', so to speak!

4 We can call on 'all those of goodwill' across the

earth. This is a very potent force. For instance,
during my healing ceremonies, I even call upon 'all
those trees of goodwill' growing down the carr where
I live!

5 Finally, we call upon the power of the angels.

The Ceremony

As we begin our healing ceremony, we direct the power we have
invoked into the work in hand by a powerful effort of will and a
steady concentration of the mind. We do this not only by
employing our own will and focus, but also via a prayer to the
angels of power to help us thus to channel the energies we have
invoked.

We then intone a prayer for the type of angel, or angels,
appropriate to the work to be present and bid them take charge
of and assist the work.

It is worth remembering, at this point, that the angels never
fail to respond to our call. Not only do we ourselves increase the
power of our work a thousandfold when we unite with the angels
in performing it, but the angels themselves find that their powers
are similarly increased. Geoffrey Hodson says, 'In all cases the
union of human and angelic consciousness and power achieves a
far greater result than is possible in the case of either working
alone.'

One of the many wonderful aspects of the angelic hierarchy
is that they can continue working with a patient or a project we
have underway, emanating, insulating, revitalizing, fostering,
directing, focusing, coordinating and protecting the healing
forces we have invoked, whilst we are only able to give the
work in hand certain and inevitably limited measurements of
our time. Their ability to remain in attendance throughout the
entire course of a project of healing, cleansing, protection,
blessing or clearing should always be utilized to the full in our
healing work. We can add to this a direction to the angels to

remain with the patient at a deeply personal and emotional level, to 'sustain the sufferers and to lift them into the conscious realization of the divine presence and of their own angelic companionship'. Geoffrey Hodson also advises us:

> We may close with a final prayer that the sufferers
> may be held close in the everlasting arms and that
> the holy angels may encompass them. We must
> always safeguard such efforts as these by a
> surrender to the divine will in everything that is
> done. We then minimise the likelihood of error
> through ignorance or misdirection of force.

From _Thus Have I Heard_

The Angel Hours

Although there are individual angels who stand guard over each hour, the angelic hours are divided into cusps or pinnacles of supernal energy which occur every three hours in divisions of three. Beginning at three o'clock in the morning, they occur at six, nine, twelve noon, three, six, nine and twelve midnight. If you can plan your ceremonies to coincide with this 'three rhythm', they will certainly gain added power from it. However, your rituals will still be extremely useful and blessed by the angels even if you are unable to comply with the angelic hours.

Finally, we need to remember that absent healing will comprise most of our task in angel healing. Very profound work is implemented on the patient's soul plane, which is where the real problem lies. In the soul state, the patient is called upon by name and escorted to the healing temple in the spiritual worlds. We carry out the necessary work before our altar, directing the angelic colours into the patient via the sacred forces within our hands and heart as if he or she stood there in front of us, and calling upon the angels in the ways that are described above.

The remainder of this chapter contains references and correspondences that I hope will be useful to you in your angel healing endeavours. The angel who is overlighting this book is
called Sabinda or Sar Binda (I am rather intrigued by the ori-
ental sound of the name!). She-he will help and protect all
those who call upon her-his wisdom and grace, particularly
those light servers who work with the methods outlined in this
book. Sar Binda offers protection, inspiration and guidance.

When people are ill, their aura is often murky and polluted.
This produces many malfunctions of the body and mind. People's
thoughts actually take shape, and flow into their aura. They even
create entities! Yes, our thoughts actually burgeon with vital life-
forms. They are like dream creatures, lovely and benign if our
thoughts are beautiful, goblinesque and crone-like if they are
not! They surround us and play out dramas in the ethers of the
life we have given them, creating 'atmosphere'. They attract
other life-forms of similar ilk. Thus, when we are sad or angry, we
can often feel the inner situation growing worse, seemingly of its
own accord. By the same token, if we are happy and humorous,
the very air around us seems to turn golden, or to bubble with
hilarity. Gifted comics attract humorous entities at will, and
build castles in the air from their configurations and mental and
emotional antics, bringing an audience under their spell.

Lively, virile, sweet-aspected thoughts charge the air in and
around our aura, leaving invigorating currents in their wake
which give us good health and a sense of wellbeing. They are like
spiritual oxygen and electricity. Negative thought-entities, on
the other hand, tend not to move on. Their gift is very different,
not a shimmer of gold but one of tacky dim tar or slime, which
clogs our mental and emotional footsteps. It builds up in our
aura, and in this specially created element, the dark entities live
and thrive – on the life energy of their host. They suck it up and
actually get very fat, sometimes so obese that they begin to push
our aura, which has the contours of a perfect egg, severely out of
shape. These breeding dark thought-forms choke the activity

of the chakras and the life forces flowing through them and through the aura, prevent the attraction of spiritual vibrations from the cosmos, and inhibit our own spontaneous negation and clearing of adverse attractions and invasion emanating from the earth and from other people.

Sometimes people secrete a deep pain-entity in their aura. It will have penetrated their defences via some profound shock or heartbreak in their present, or even a previous, existence. The pain-entity will remain dormant until the person concerned tries to move in a life direction which will overcome the domination of this astral creature formulated from their pain, shame, guilt or fear. Suddenly alert to the situation, the pain-demon flares up, taking on the dimensions of a great overarching giant, threatening to overwhelm its human host with a world of suffering even worse and more terrifying than the trauma of their original experience. It is lying, of course – but it is a very accomplished liar! And so people settle in terror back into their old mindsets, where at least they feel safe, if also thoroughly miserable and oppressed.

We can see how necessary it is for the angels to step in and take matters in hand concerning scenarios of this kind. Without them, left entirely to our own devices, we would have no hope of routing such enemies; but the angels know how to rescue us, and to place the sword of our own emancipation in our hand.

Named Angels

I offer here a selection of named angels to help you in your work. Whilst it is always good to be able to sound an angelic name and to chant it, it is also important not to tie ourselves to a rigid system of correspondences, or think in terms of cataloguing when we consider angels! Such concepts have nothing to do with the reality of the limitless, boundless angelic life-stream, which is an expression of spiritual freedom.

The named angels given are ready to lend their support in

specific circumstances, but, again, we must remind ourselves not to think in terms of limitation. There are so many rapturously wonderful angels whose names we do not know, whose existence we have not dreamt of. Think of the Angel of the Breath of Silence, or the Angel of the Fragrance of the Rose, or the Angel of the Beauty of the Moon. How about the Angel of the Laughter in Water? She could reveal a dimension to you whose secrets your imagination has never touched upon.

Are you feeling jaded, brittle minded, dried up inside? Call on the Angel of Dew! Do you need to encourage concerted effort, harmonious unity, among work colleagues so that a project may be brought to fruition? Summon the Angel of the Bees! Always remember that we can be as creative and far-ranging as we like in our concepts of the angelic hierarchy and their ability to heal our life situations as well as our illnesses. Our imaginings will never outdo the angels!

Each angel encompasses both genders, so when you call on the named angels, they will attend you in the gender which most suits the healing operation they undertake (they may also use their androgynous form).

Afriel

Call on this angel in the treatment of children, and the inner child residing within each one of us. Afriel imparts youth and vitality, and reminds us that old age is actually nothing more than a thought-form to which we subscribe. Afriel brings rejuvenation and vigour to our physical and subtle organs.

Akriel

The Angel of Memory. Pray to this luminary when a memory needs sharpening.

Anahita

This angel is a caretaker of the Earth and her fecundity. Pray to her to heal the earth, or any part of it which has become barren.

Angels of Water

These are traditionally known as Azariel, Tharsis, Michael, Gabriel and Nahaliel. They protect, cleanse and heal all bodies of water on earth. The angels of the rivers are Trsiel, Enki and Dara. We can invoke their powers and benediction when we want to bring healing to the waters of the earth – a task that the angels will delight in and bless us for.

Armaita

This gracious one fosters harmonious, balanced, cooperative relationships with others. She presides over Truth.

Balthial

An angel who helps us to overcome jealousy, and feelings of inadequacy, bitterness and resentment.

Barbelo

An 'educator' angel. She will uplift and inspire your patients to think more in terms of spiritual values. She sheds a golden efful-gence onto life's ups and downs, so that the breath and beneficence of Divine Spirit may be sensed through them, leading us home to the light of our eternal selves.

Cathetel

We can pray to this guardian angel of gardens when we wish to invoke healing for a struggling or infested garden. Dorothea is the guardian spirit of gardens.

Chamuel

Call on Chamuel to inspire tolerance and to soften harsh, critical, antagonistic attitudes. Chamuel helps us to love and to forgive ourselves, and to let go of a judgemental outlook on life, our own failings, and those of other people.

Charoum
The Angel of Silence. For patients who need the dynamic of peace both within and without, we can summon the blessing of both Charoum and Valoel (*see* above). Charoum blesses the art of listening and teaches us to set a guard over our tongue. 'There is a mighty power in silence,' say the angels. How often in life do we feel pressured, really against our will, to say something, to respond with some remark, when it would be better not to do so, but rather to keep a gracious silence? The colour of silence is pure white, pure light, and those who can be graciously silent reveal themselves thereby as old initiates. They have mastered the art of silence. Let us remember the option of silence, with all its poise, dignity and peace.

Elemiah
This angel blesses the depths of our self-awareness. Call on this radiant one to illuminate blind spots, blinkeredness and ignorance or distorted ideas of self.

Gabriel
A great archangel of joy and beauty. Enfold your patients in Gabriel's gift of radiant happiness.

Gavreel
The Peace-Maker Angel, Gavreel resolves situations of enmity and conflict into forgiveness, acceptance and peace. As well as helping us to make peace with our enemies, Gavreel fosters mental and emotional balance and brings the balm of peace to troubled minds. Those enduring destructive stress or otherwise in need of equilibrium can invoke Gavreel and his merciful powers.

Gazardiel
The Angel of the Rising Sun, Gazardiel protects children and all young, tender, growing things. When patients long to feel the promise of new beginnings, of a tender enfoldment in newfound

innocence after experiencing the sense of its loss, or stands in need of forces of renewal, awakening and a rebirth of enlightenment in life, teach them to face the rising sun each morning and invoke the blithe, radiant, tender Gazardiel.

Haamiah
An angel of truth and integrity. When we withhold honesty from ourselves or others, it harms our soul. A mist covers our feelings and our relationships with others – a confusing, distressing mist that makes everything, life's normal dynamics, seem stressful and traumatic. If you have lost sight of your own truth and you feel the resultant pull away from your centre, your integrity, call this angel into your field of spiritual vision with a sincere prayer for help. She will restore you to yourself.

Hael
An angel of art and beauty who inspires mercy and kindness to flourish in human hearts. When a patient is in need of mercy and kindness, either as virtues within themselves or as blessings in their lives, we call on Hael.

Hahaiah
This beneficent one ignites and fosters the beautiful flame of happy, positive and loving thoughts, feelings and impulses in our mind, heart and soul.

Haniel
Haniel teaches us to experience romantic love from a standpoint of poise, balance and sanity. Although most of us want wildness, poetry and passion in our deepest love-affairs, these elements have to be kept in creative rather than destructive mode. Their keynote must be love, rather than desire. Haniel shows us how to achieve a proper perspective by combining personal love with unconditional love, and unconditional love with the appropriate degree of responsibility to self. She teaches us to embrace

wisdom, insight and stability whilst we enjoy the euphoria of being in love.

Hariel
The Angel of companion and domestic animals. He brings healing and protection to pets and farm animals, and shelters them from abuse.

Iahel
The Angel of Meditation. Pray to this Chieftain of the Halls of Boundless Light for depth, clarity and guidance along the path of truth in your meditations.

Isda
The Angel of Nourishment. We can invoke her for nourishment on every level, and to help those who suffer from a misunderstanding of nourishment which has taken deep root in their psyche, so that they are underweight or overweight. Baglis works with this angel. Isda shows us how to nourish ourselves with self-love (different from selfishness), so that expressions of undernourishment or overnourishment become unnecessary.

Israfel
Israfel, the beautiful Angel of Music, is the personification of healing. Rhythmically, lyrically, harmoniously, he regenerates, resurrects and renews with his exquisite art which enchants and transfigures the soul and releases the spiritual fire within her. Call on Israfel when you sense the presence of broken harmony and broken rhythm, either in yourself, your patients, or the environment.

Itkal
This luminary has dominion over cooperation and the formation of loving bonds between people. She nurtures the establishment of harmonious relationships. Omniel, Mihr and

Itkal work together, and can be summoned together with prayer and invocation.

Jophiel
This great angel liberates our minds and our outlook from the bonds of programming and conditioning attached to sources which are not in harmony with the wisdom of our soul. He brings us emancipation, enlightenment, and the courage of open-mindedness.

Lazai
Call on this 'holy angel of God' to heal inflammation and heat-producing maladies.

Maion
The Angel of Self-Discipline. This bright spirit holds up the ideal of wise self-regulation and denial of the demands and dominion of the lower self, but counsels against harshness. She reminds us that self-flagellation can be a form of indulgence! Attune yourself to this angel to learn the gentle but persistent art of self-governance.

Mihr
The Angel of Friendship, Mihr can be summoned to heal rifts between friends and our general relationships with others; and also to heal an inability to make friends.

Mtniel
The Guardian Angel of Wild Animals, Mtniel helps us to heal our animal brethren.

Nemamiah
Angel of Just Causes. We invoke Nemamiah to heal an injustice, especially one dealt out to the frail and the vulnerable, and to bless any worthy cause our work might lead us to undertake.

Nin Khursag

As Lady of the Mountain, we pray to Nin Khursag for stability, steadfastness, firmness and the strength to endure.

Omniel

This angel fosters our connectedness with one another. He lifts us into Divine Oneness and heals our tendency towards isolation of self. Those suffering from loneliness, from autism, from imbalances in the ego, will benefit from the healing influences of this shining one.

Orifiel

Angel of the Wilderness. When we wish to heal and protect wild places in nature, we summon the stewardship of Orifiel.

Rehael

This Son of the Flame fosters respect for parents and for wisdom arising from ancient sources, not only human but from all the world of Nature and her many kingdoms. When a person is disconnected from their source, when children (or indeed adults) have no respect for their parents, we call in this angel as troubleshooter.

Rhamiel

This sacred being is the Angel of Compassion. Her wing-beats form spiritual waves of compassion, empathy, mercy, sympathy. When a patient needs to receive these beautiful qualities, or to express them, the angel Rhamiel is at hand to help.

Sachael

Sachael is the Angel of the Waters of the Soul. She teaches us what water really is in the higher realms. The soul itself is actually formed from an exalted form of ethereal water. She fosters our intuitive powers and brings to us an awareness and understanding of our deepest feelings. She teaches us how to perfectly reflect the still flame of the spirit so that we can claim our highest birthright. She releases pressure and disturbance from the unconscious realms, and makes clear and pure any area of the waters of our soul that have grown murky and unwholesome.

Shekinah and Brigid

These two mighty female angels are beings of the brilliant light of the Ineffable. Brigid is the Bride, the Immortal Daughter of Goddess-God. Shekinah is the angelic aspect of Brigid, highest among angels, consort to Archangel Michael. Both of these golden ones, Beings of Inconceivable Fire, bring a burgeoning abundance of healing to humankind of body, mind and spirit. They teach our souls the Dance of Life. Call on them in any and every healing situation.

Shemael

Shemael fosters the upwelling of gratitude in the human heart. When these springs have run dry or become choked, depression and a feeling of disgust with life is the inevitable result. Energy does not replenish itself, and a person may put on weight in an attempt to draw mental and physical energy from food and the act of eating. When life seems grey, desolate and grief-stricken, it is difficult to feel gratitude for the experience of it. Therefore, we treat depressive, world-weary patients with Shemael's gentle, compassionate gifts, so that the deep wellsprings of the spirit may be renewed.

Sofiel

Another angel of the garden. Sofiel has particular guardianship over fruits and vegetables, helping them to flourish and keep healthy. Sofiel is also a wonderful grounding angel, and will reconnect sick and depleted mortals to vital earth energies. When you sense a blockage or a lack of the upflowing forces from the earth in a patient's aura, call on Sofiel.

Tabris

This angel is set over free will, self-determination and indepen-
dence of choice. We invoke Tabris when we need help to lift
ourselves out of a stalemate or stuck situation and seek to become
aware of creative alternatives. Remember Colopatiron, the angel
who comes to unlock the prison gate. One can imagine many uses
for the beneficent powers of these two luminaries in any therapeutic
practice. Tabris and Colpatiron work together. They also grant
mortals the necessary patience and endurance to wait quietly
and alertly for that moment when their release comes.

Trgiaob (Trr-gia-ob)

The angel protector of birds of the wilderness. The name of this
angel is pronounced rather like a birdcall! Try to get that fluting,
chirruping rhythm with which birds sing when you sound her-his
name, and repeat it just as birds delight in the repetitive tempo
of their song (the final syllable 'ob' rises pertly in tone). You can
summon Trgiaob to protect all wild birds from disease, abuse,
reduction in numbers, pollution and the destruction of their
habitat, and to heal individual wild birds. Let Trgiaob also foster
within your soul the love of birdsong.

When you concentrate on it with a rapt, spiritually listening
heart, embracing each note with every sense open and atten-
tive, birdsong will carry you directly into the world of the angels.
The angels share a link with birds and birdsong which earthliness cannot sully, and the chaotic noise of our modern
civilization cannot silence. It will always be magical, and indeed
it is magic of the highest order. If you want to enter the fairy
worlds, the angelic worlds, whilst still on earth, one certain way
to do so is to open your inner ear to birdsong. (I must relate that,
whilst sitting at my desk beside an open door into my garden
and trying out the sound of Trgiaob's name as I was writing the
above passage, a cuckoo (my favourite bird, the messenger of
Goddess), flew into my garden and, perching on a tree, sat and
sang a cascade of its mellifluent, bell-like notes for quite a few

minutes before flying off! This is especially unusual, as the date is 22 June, and in this area I have never heard a cuckoo sing after the 21st of the month. Moreover, there has been a scarcity of cuckoos for a couple of years in the part of Lincolnshire where I live, and this was the first of the year (and no doubt the last) for me. In past years, when they were less rare, I always heard them calling in the woods at the bottom of the long lane that winds past my house; but no cuckoo has ever before actually visited my garden, nor have I ever actually seen one! I was left with the distinct feeling that I had encountered a spirit visitation in bird form. I hope this encourages you to get closely in touch with Trgiaob!)

Valoel
Valoel is the sublime Angel of Peace. We can call on this great one to bless us with a serene mind, a tranquil heart and peaceful dreams. We can also ask Valoel to bring the balm of healing peace to an aggravated situation or relationship.

The Virtues
We call on The Virtues when we need a transformation of conditions or circumstances. They are a high order of angels whose principal duty is to work miracles on earth.

Vohu Manah ('good thought')
This wonderful angel blesses and uplifts our thoughts and our thought-sphere (the vessel which generates, contains, attracts, reflects and distributes our thoughts). All patients with a negative, anxious or pessimistic outlook, or with angry, conceited or otherwise inharmonious thought-energy, need to be brought before Vohu Manah.

When we think of the maxim of the angels – that the three great tasks of angel healers are to educate, to cleanse, and to attune – we can see how Vohu Manah assists us in all three. Our first directive in educating our patients must be to encourage

them to create within themselves a triumphal march of good
thought, to transmute the harmful accumulation of dark
thought-entities they unknowingly harbour in their auric fields.
To cleanse them of this poisonous psychic material is essential;
and the attunement of the subtle bodies of each patient to the
spiritual emanations of the stars and to the inflow of angelic consciousness with all the blessing, inspiration and healing it brings,
cannot be achieved without the attuning power of the positive
vibrations of 'good thought'.

The Voices

The Gnostics described these enigmatic angels as angelic entities
inhabiting the Treasury of Light. From this Treasury they have
gifts to bring us, gifts of inner counselling, guidance, enlightenment, comfort and inspiration. When we are weary, getting
nowhere, when we seem to have turned blind and deaf to all
spiritual direction, when we or our patients seem to come up
against a brick wall, then we call on The Voices. Tradition tells
us there are seven Voices. They have passed into folklore as the
Seven Whistlers (birds with a melancholy call, such as plovers,
curlews or lapwings, who foretell tragedy, especially on the sea)
and the Seven Wish Hounds (baying voices who also foretell
death). It is interesting to note that folklore is full of doom and
gloom concerning The Voices, when actually they bring life and
hope! Sometimes they do issue a warning, but only with the
expectation of averting the threatening incident, not for the
pleasure of prophesying woe! Perhaps the real reason lies in the
influence of established political and religious bodies, who were
careful to frighten people concerning The Voices because they
preferred the populace not to be in direct touch with the Divine
themselves, fearing what might happen (to their power and all
its privileges) if individual minds were not held under the sway
of a common authority.

Vrihaspati

Guardian of hymns, invocations and prayers, this venerable one is said to be 'first-born in the highest Heaven of supreme light'. We can call on Vrihaspati to bless our prayers and invocations, and help us to formulate new ones that are beautiful and effective, and which please the angels. Don't be inhibited when you feel the touch of Vrihaspati's inspiration. Whilst writing an invocation for a patient who needed more magnetism in her aura, I received the suggestion that I should evoke the mantle of the Angel of the Moon to enfold her, and surround her with 'the music of the moon'. It seemed to work quite well!

Yadael

This angel will assist us in our ceremonial rites. Yadael is a guardian angel of the gates of the north wind, and will protect the angelic altar and all influences coming to it from the sacred direction of the north. The angels of the four cardinal points are: Archangel Uriel in the east, Archangel Michael in the south, Archangel Raphael in the west, and Archangel Gabriel in the north. You might like to call on these archangels for protection and blessings for your angelic altar, turning to face each direction as you call.

Yahoel ('beauty of God')

One of the great angels, Yahoel guides the leaders of humanity. Pray to this mighty one if you are working to heal a political or environmental situation which hangs on the making of wise decisions by those in positions of leadership.

Yahriel

Invoke this angel when you need to heal a condition locked in the subconscious. Yahriel holds dominion over the moon, who is queen of the subconscious realms.

Yusamin

This shining being may be invoked when we need the blessing of fertility at any level – mentally, emotionally or physically. Yusamin is an aspect of our well-known Samandiriel.

Zeruel ('arm of God')

When you need to invoke the quality of strength, of will, of body, of purpose, strength for the aura or the strength of courage, endurance and resilience, call on Zeruel, an angel 'set over strength'.

Zlar

When you need spiritual insight and penetrative perception, call on this mighty being, 'one of the company of glorious and benevolent angels' who reveals secret wisdom.

Zoroel

A powerful healing angel, able to overcome the dominion of even the lordliest amongst the disease and pain elementals (entities which create and hold in place the etheric patterns and systems which bring into being, feed and perpetuate disease and pain).

Zotiel ('little one of God')

This angel, from the order of cherubs, can be invoked to bring comfort to fearful children, or to adults who are very insecure and timid. Zotiel is one of the 'whispering angels' – angels who bring healing and reassurance to patients by a constant whispering in the ear of the wisdom and goodness of Divine Spirit, and of the unfailing love and protection of the angels.

Zumech

This 'most holy angel of God' will bless your angel altar, and all your healing ceremonies, with the potent, blissful magic of the heavenly realms.

Zuphlas

The great angel protector of trees, who can be called upon to heal and bless individual trees, copses and woodland, or the great forests of the world. We hear the grandeur of Zuphlas's music when the wind is in the treetops, or when we stand and listen, in utter stillness of soul, within the depths of winter or summer woods. Zuphlas is eager to work with us. If you are seeking to bring wisdom and angel blessings to a political assembly that will make decisions about the environment, call on Zuphlas to descend upon and inspire those who will receive her-his guidance.

Zuriel ('my rock is God')

We can call on this prince of angels to help us overcome the mindsets and stumbling blocks that bar our way forward (to be brutally frank, Zuriel is known as a 'curer of the stupidity in man'!). We seek Zuriel's help in illuminating dim spiritual sight and opening spiritually deaf ears. Of course, we should always be careful to convey Zuriel's blessing as a free gift from the heart, rather than with the thought of replacing a person's individual viewpoint with our own!

Remember, it must be stressed that there is no need to call on specifically named angels if you prefer not to. You can always invoke the angels of peace, the angels of compassion, the angels of courage, etc.

Chakra Healing

The healing implements of the soul and the tools of communion that we use to help us in our task of angel healing (*see* Chapters Two and Three) may also be applied specifically in the case of difficulty at the level of any particular chakra. For instance, if you or your patient are fearful and the world seems dark and threatening, this would indicate a need to overcome the challenge of the base chakra. Using the corresponding image when you prepare your healing ceremonies and invocations and when you sit for healing meditations may be of real assistance. Of course, the implements are valuable in themselves, without forming part of a system, which should never be rigidly applied. The following is only a guideline.

1 The Rose	Smell	Base Chakra
2 The Breath	Taste	Sacral Chakra
3 The Star	Sight	Solar Plexus
4 The Chalice	Touch	Heart Chakra
5 The Silence	Hearing	Throat Chakra
6 The Rainbow Bridge	Sixth Sense	Third Eye
7 Meditation	Cosmic Consciousness	Full Moon Crown Chakra
	Balance	Unicorn's Horn Crown Chakra
8 Meditation in the Rose Temple	Mind-in-the-Heart ('Nous')	Earth Chakra (Hands and Feet)

The eighth chakra tool (relating to the earth chakra) reflects the seventh chakra tool (relating to the crown chakra), and is therefore also Meditation, but with its magenta quality emphasized (symbolized by the rose temple).

The Archangels and the Chakras

The archangels and the chakras share a certain correspondence, but, again, we must not limit ourselves to any particular system. However, when we are implementing our healing services and are treating our patients with beautiful hues from the angelic

colour spectrum playing in and over the rainbow chalice in the
heart, it is reassuring to ask the relevant archangels to monitor
and bless the healing work taking place on the chakras, and to
seal them afterwards. The following list gives the traditional
associations.

The Chakra and Archangel Correspondences

BASE CHAKRA
Archangel Sandalphon
The Earth Angel
Archangel Camael
Archangel Cassiel
Brigid

SACRAL CHAKRA
Archangel Chamuel
Archangel Gabriel
Archangel Haniel

SOLAR PLEXUS CHAKRA
Archangel Uriel
Archangel Jophiel
Archangel Michael

HEART CHAKRA
Archangel Raphael
Archangel Chamuel
Archangel Shekinah
Archangel Haniel
Archangel Michael
Brigid
Merlin's Secret Queen

THROAT CHAKRA
Archangel Michael
Archangel Haniel
Brigid

BROW CHAKRA
Archangel Gabriel
Archangel Jophiel
Archangel Raphael
Archangel Uriel

CROWN CHAKRA
Archangel Gabriel
Brigid
Merlin's Secret Queen
Archangel Zadkiel
Archangel Michael
Archangel Shekinah
Archangel Asariel

EARTH CHAKRA
Brigid
Merlin's Secret Queen
Archangel Gabriel
Archangel Zadkiel
Archangel Cassiel
Archangel Sandalphon
The Earth Angel

CHAPTER EIGHT

CRYSTAL HEALING
WEBS

Angels and crystals share a natural affinity because crystals are manifestations of matter exalted and purified until they independently radiate the spirit of beauty and perfection. The molecular complexity of crystals allows angelic consciousness to resonate with their vibrations and even to dwell therein. We can, therefore, use crystals to assist us to contact the angelic realm, and to receive amplified healing emanations from it, due to the streamlining effect of the crystals upon these emanations, which helps them to penetrate deep into earthly dimensions and sustains them in a highly functioning state.

Crystals have individual consciousness which the angels uplift and harmonize with their own. We need to remember, however, that when a crystal comes to us, it has been mined. It has been harshly and unceremoniously torn from its native environment, and it may well be in a state of disorientation and shock. We can pray to the healing angels, and to Archangel Cassiel, who has rulership over precious and semiprecious stones, to soothe the trauma the crystal has suffered. At the same time as we offer the prayer, we hold the crystal within the caressing petals of the rose in the heart, and shine the light of the star into the depths of the stone. We also send a prayer and a blessing, via the healing angels and Archangel Cassiel, to the crystal's place of origin, the mother-source, which will feel the loss of the mined crystal. In this way, we restore the spiritual pattern to which our crystal belonged before it was removed, and in which it was working. That work can then continue unhindered, and the bilateral signals of distress and confusion are eased into peace and silence.

All crystals must be cleansed regularly, but when we work with crystals to heal ourselves or others, it is vital that they are thoroughly purified both before and after each healing session. Generally, a quick wash (no more than a second or two) under the flow of the cold tap is all that is required. When we are working with patients who suffer from a serious illness, or whose energy is very heavy and blocked, the crystals require a more elaborate cleansing ritual. The quickest way is to place them in a glass bowl of spring water, add a large spoonful of apple cider vinegar (one of the varieties produced from whole apples) and leave them to soak for a few hours, preferably outside in the sunlight, although this is not essential. Avoid using tap water to fill the glass bowl. Tap water contains negative energy patterns because of the chemicals used to clean it, which should not be passed on to the crystals. These negative patterns do not affect crystals when the stream from the cold tap is used for a few seconds to cleanse them, but they do take their toll if the crystals are immersed in tap water for any length of time.

When you remove the crystals, dry them, and hold them in the palm of your left hand. Create the form of the star in your heart. Say, 'I bless these crystals in the name of the Divine Spirit, and dedicate them to the highest good. I ask the angels of the Divine Spirit to cleanse them of all consciousness which is not their own, or is not that with which I programme them.' Let the light from the star in your heart shine out over the crystals, and in imagination place them in the golden-white glow of your heart, where there is a cave for their safekeeping. Your crystals are now blessed, dedicated and cleansed, and are ready to be programmed.

Strictly speaking, it is really only possible to programme clear quartz. However, I find that other varieties do seem to respond to the first part of the following programming process.

- Cup the crystal in your left palm, hold it to your heart, and intone your patient's name slowly, three times.

- Speak to the crystal (it is a centre of consciousness) and make a clearly worded request that it should bring healing to your patient (always refer to your patient by name).

- Ask for specific healing ('May the healing power go to the liver, the bowel, the heart, the stomach, the nervous system, etc., to restore [the patient's name]').

If you are working with clear quartz crystal, continue with the second part of the process.

- Decide clearly which qualities you wish to be programmed into the crystal (or crystals).

- Radiating it from your own heart-centre, focusing it with your mind into the crystal, flood the crystal with the particular quality in which you wish your patient to be bathed (vitality, love, healing from the angels, peace and calm, consolation, courage, cheerfulness, etc.).

- Let this be done, not so much at the mental level, but as an act of illumined imagination arising from the heart, so that you really feel the quality with which you are imbuing the crystal. If you have difficulty, remember to call on the angels for help. Act out the emotion, as if you were on stage demonstrating it, and the angels will fill the vessel you thereby create with the appropriate 'note' or feeling.

There are seven crystal healing webs which I have found effective in the practice of angel healing. Of course, if you make a particular study of crystals, you may wish to formulate many more. The seven simple webs that I use are given below. Crystal healing webs are laid out around a patient reclining on the floor or on a mattress and some of the crystals are actually placed on the patient's body.

It is a good idea to use angel affirmations whilst patients are undergoing treatment in a web. (Treatment usually continues for about half an hour.) Prior to the beginning of the treatment, explain to the patient that the web will link them with the angels, and that your voice becomes the voice of their own wise angelic self speaking to them from the realms of the soul. Play some beautiful music, let the patient absorb the energy and peace of the web, then turn down the music gradually until all is silent. Allow the patient to enter the silence. Then repeat the angel affirmation for them three times. Before beginning the affirmation, intone the patient's name aloud three times. Whilst you are doing so, send out a silent request to the angels that they transform your voice into a healing channel for the patient concerned.

Angel Crystal Healing Web – Raphael

This web is linked to Archangel Raphael.

A clear quartz crystal point is placed above the head.

A rutile quartz is placed at the level of the crown chakra.

A clear quartz is placed on the third eye chakra.

A green aventurine is placed at the base of the brain chakra.

A citrine is placed on the throat chakra.

An angelite stone is held in each hand.

An amethyst and a rose quartz are placed upon the heart-centre.

A smoky quartz is placed at the base chakra.

A clear quartz point is placed beneath each foot.

AFFIRMATION FOR THE RAPHAEL WEB

Archangel Raphael, I feel your healing presence, and the presence of your healing angels. I am healed. I am healed. I am healed. I am whole in mind. I am whole in spirit. I am whole in body. I am healed. Thank you for your healing touch.

Of course, you can adjust these words to your patient's particular condition.

Angel Crystal Healing Web – Rainbow

This web balances the chakras. Although the colours of the chakras do not entirely equate with the colours of the rainbow, there is a correspondence between them.

An amethyst, red calcite and a rose quartz are placed below the feet.

A red jasper and a smoky quartz are placed at the level of the base chakra.

A carnelian is placed on the sacral chakra.

A citrine is placed on the solar plexus chakra.

A green aventurine, morganite and a rose quartz are placed in a triangle over the heart-centre.

A blue lace agate and a rutile quartz are placed on the throat chakra.

A lapiz lazuli is placed on the third eye chakra.

Three amethysts are placed in a triangle over the crown chakra.

Place a clear quartz point above this triangle.

AFFIRMATION FOR THE RAINBOW WEB

Great angels of the rainbow, I sense your healing
power streaming down upon me in an exquisite
play of rainbow colours. I make my solemn
promise to you to absorb this healing in full, and
to stay true to its beautiful vibrations in my daily
life. I am strong in the light! I am strong in the
light! I am strong in the light, and the light never
fails me and is always with me. Thank you for your
healing embrace. You hold me always in the
rhythm and harmony of Goddess-God's unbroken
peace. All is well.

The three angel crystal healing webs that follow are the simplest
of all. They each make use of only one type of crystal.

Rose Quartz Crystal Healing Web – Archangel Chamuel

Place a piece of rose quartz upon each chakra, one above the
head, one in each hand, and one below each foot.

You can adapt this ceremony for any condition which is
caused by emotional neediness or deprivation.

Burn a few drops of rose oil in a censer, and rub a drop or two
into the wrists and the third eye of your patients. Ask them to
apply the oil to the heart-centre. (Remember that you will need
a carrier oil, such as almond, for all aromatherapy oils except
lavender. The ratio is 2.5 per cent essential oil to 97.5 per cent
carrier oil. This is achieved by dividing the number of millilitres
of a bottle of carrier oil in two to calculate the number of drops
of essential oil you should add to it; so for a 12ml bottle of carrier
oil, you would add six drops of essential oil to create a safe blend,
or ten drops to a 20ml bottle of carrier oil, etc.)

Summon the archangel Chamuel, and the other angels you have chosen to help your patients, to oversee the ceremony and bring blessings, healing and freedom from limitation to the soul. Speak this affirmation for them:

> I now contemplate the presence of the perfect rose, blush-pink as sunrise, deep in the innermost chamber of my heart. The tender fragrant petals enfold my consciousness, and I am taken by Archangel Chamuel into the essence of the mystic bloom, which is the temple of the rose. In this softly radiant temple I am safe, and loved by the angels. I give my uttermost permission to Archangel Chamuel, to all the angels invoked for my healing, and to the angels of the rose quartz that surrounds me, to attune my body, my heart, and all my chakras to the rose ray of Divine Love.
>
> Within this sacred rose temple is the magic circle of Divine Spirit's infinite love and beauty, and I am centred in it. I now unite my soul with the rays of peace and joy, goodness and love which shine on me from the heart of Goddess-God. I join in the angels' perpetual song of happiness, harmony and bliss. I know that I am cherished and infinitely loved, held and protected forever and for always in the heart of Goddess-God.
>
> All that used to manifest as unhappiness and distress within me is subsumed in this great golden current of Love. I am enfolded in the fragrance of the rose and the Angel of the Rose bears me up in everlasting arms. I enter the deep silence of Goddess-God, and breathe in God's harmony and rhythm perpetually. All is well.

Clear Quartz Crystal Healing Web – Archangel Michael

Place a piece of clear crystal quartz upon each chakra and one in each hand; place a clear crystal quartz point above the head, and one below each foot.

You can programme and imbue clear quartz crystal with any healing property or quality you choose. I have selected an angelic affirmation for the relief of depression and inertia. Although tranquillity is needed by depressive patients, one of the truly vital components of their healing treatment is to get their subtle energies moving. Depression will not be relieved until this process is initiated. We call on Archangel Michael and his angels of joy, courage, faith and vitality for patients who undertake this crystal web treatment.

You may like to use rosemary or citrus oil for this ceremony. The carrier oil containing the citrus or rosemary drops should be rubbed into the palms of the hands and the soles of the feet, into the solar plexus centre and into the base of the brain chakra. The base of the spine centre should also be treated. The oil is not actually applied to this chakra. Instead, the piece of clear crystal quartz which has been placed at the base of the spine is anointed and returned to its station.

Once you have invoked the angels, intone the following affirmation.

> Archangel Michael dwells in the right ventricle of my heart, and Archangel Shekinah dwells in the left. Their wingbeats pulsate the magical happiness of golden sunlight from the angelic realms throughout my brain and body, throughout each of my chakras, throughout my aura. This golden sunlight, sparkling with vivacity, enables me to achieve a state of perpetual happiness.

> I realize that the shadows of fear, anxiety, hostility,

hopelessness, despair, exhaustion and misery that cloud my vision are unreal. I now dispel these shadows with the golden radiance of truth. Lightly, with winged feet, I ascend the spiritual mountaintop and look out with wonder into the limitless vistas of God's eternality, golden with happiness.

The entire universe is ringing with the loving laughter of the angels of faith and the angels of joy. The angels of vitality add their note to the choir, bringing a flush of orange into the golden picture which fills my centres with a fiery zest and leaping energy. Now the angels of courage join the rejoicing throng, great winged man-lions, some mighty and feminine.

My heart opens, and they fill me until I overflow with the exalting warmth of their measureless courage. Dancing in the wondrous flames of the love of the angels and of Divine Spirit, I summon an irresistible shaft of willpower and here and now I banish all negative and ill-willed forces from my consciousness and from my environment. I enter the rhythm and harmony of God and all is well.

Amethyst Crystal Healing Web –
Archangel Zadkiel

Place an amethyst upon each chakra, one in each hand, one below each foot, and a chevron amethyst above the head.

For this healing ceremony, you can use lavender oil in an incense burner. Rub a little of the oil onto the wrists of the patient, and onto their third eye chakra.

Intone the following affirmation at the appropriate time.

Archangel Zadkiel, descend into my heart and be
with me. I see your Violet Flame take form and

chase through every amethyst that surrounds me,
encompassing me in a circle of your beautiful
violet light.

(In this instance, it is better if the patient herself repeats the following invocation after you.)

'I AM a being of violet fire!

I AM the purity God Desires!'

Let this be affirmed three times, or more if the patient desires it.

You can be a little more flexible with the rose quartz and the clear quartz healing webs. Use the first for any illness or condition which seems to have its roots in a lack of security or deprivation of love and where the dis-ease in the patient appears to be flowing from a distressed emotional body. The clear quartz web is eminently programmable and can be used for any condition or illness. The onus here is on you as the guiding healer, because it will depend on your clarity of thought in deciding exactly what you are going to ask of the crystals on behalf of your patients, and your emotional clarity and flow in programming the crystals with the relevant qualities. You may find that you yourself need some healing before you begin to try to help others. This is usually the case. We take the time and care we need for ourselves without stinting, so that we can give of our best to our patients.

The little affirmation ceremonies that you prepare for your patients, and intone for them as they receive treatment in a crystal healing web, can be given to them so that they can continue the treatment themselves at home (with or without the web). Teach them how to make a simple angelic altar, and to sit before it in meditation with the angels, even if for just a few moments, every day. Teach them how to cleanse their aura, chakras and environment, how to root themselves into the earth energies, and how to protect themselves with the circle of white light or the pillar of white light (our angel wings). Choose the quickest, simplest methods, or your advice will generally go unheeded!

Of course, whilst the patients work on themselves at home, you will continue the absent healing ceremonies on their behalf until they return for treatment, or until the designated period for the healing comes to an end. As you work on your absent healing ceremonies, don't be surprised if occasionally the angels give you guidance through your intuition to alter and modify them. It is true that we are aiming for stability in our healing endeavours, and constant chopping and changing is not helpful. However, if you are certain that the impulse for change is coming from the angels rather than from something restless in your nature, put it into effect immediately.

Some suggestions for the healing ceremonies follow. Before you use anything you have compiled in this respect, or whether you choose to implement the rituals given, always ask your patients to read through the material carefully to make sure that there is nothing in it to which they object. After all, you are programming their psychic centres, and their full permission must be consulted and granted. This is essential procedure. If we neglect it, the angels will not work with us, and our healing efforts will result in humiliation and confusion.

Rose Quartz and Amethyst Crystal Healing Web

A variant of the rose quartz healing web is the rose quartz and amethyst healing web. To lay it out, just place a piece of amethyst alongside each rose quartz crystal in the pattern described above. This creates the rose-amethyst or orchid ray, which brings inspiration and soul serenity as its gifts. We summon the Angel of Peace for this ceremony as well as the angels of love. It can be used as a treatment for those patients

who suffer from anxiety, insecurity, insomnia, agitation and nervousness. You might like to use chamomile, lavender and rose oil
in a blend for this crystal healing web, applying it as previously
described. Use the following affirmation.

> The angels of peace and the angels of love attune my
> soul to the soul of the universe. I grow wings of the
> spirit and soar with the angels high above the limita-
> tions and hindrances of the earth plane.

> I sing the Song Celestial, and my heart is filled with
> peace and goodness, infinite joy, calm and beauty. My
> soul blends with the presence of Goddess-God in a
> majestic rainbow of spiritual fulfilment, and the magic
> circle of divine love encompasses me and protects me
> always. I live and move and have my being in a golden
> dream of peace and soul serenity for all time.

Crystal Triangulation – The Angel of the Golden Pyramid

This particular ceremony has been adapted to treat heart conditions, although it may be applied for the treatment of any illness.

The patient sits on a chair, keeping the back supported but
straight. Place a citrine in a triangle form around him or her by
setting one beside each foot, so making the base of the flat
pyramid, and one behind the chair in line with the head, which
is its apex. Play soothing music, as usual, to allow the patient to
relax and absorb the crystal energies of the triangulation. Then
turn down the music gradually until it is inaudible, allow the
patient to enter the silence for a few minutes, and intone the following affirmation.

> The Angel of the Golden Pyramid is with me and
> blesses me. She stands at the very pinnacle of the
> golden pyramid that I see rising up before me, shining

with a bright flood of angelic gold. She holds a golden ball of this energy in her hands. She holds it forth, and its miraculous golden light flows down the pyramid into my heart and my whole cardiovascular system, gently but irresistibly cleansing, restoring, unblocking, strengthening and healing and bringing into balance all that needs to be healed.

Now the golden orb of light enters my heart, carrying the angel within it. I am restored, protected and healed. I am restored, protected and healed. I am restored, protected and healed.

Finish by saying, 'Enter into the silence. Enter into the deep harmony and rhythm of Goddess-God.' Allow the patient a few minutes to absorb this.

Ask the patient to clearly visualize each step of the ceremony as you relate it (allow time to do this by pausing between each sentence or phrase as the ceremony unfolds), and ask him or her to say the last three sentences of the affirmation with you. Then thank the Angel of the Golden Pyramid, and also the other angels that you will have chosen and invoked to preside over all the healing ceremonies you provide for the patient in question.

Important Points

- All crystals used in these rituals must be blessed, dedicated, cleansed and programmed or semi-programmed (see above) before use.
- After use, they must be thoroughly purified before being used again (for the same patient).
- If you use them for a different patient, the blessing, dedicating, cleansing and programming ritual must be adapted and enacted anew for that patient.

- When you are treating one patient for any length of time, it is a good idea to repeat the entire crystal ritual once a month.

- To reiterate, the cleansing of crystals is undertaken before and after use each time, even for absent healing ceremonies.

- Angelite is weakened by water. To clean this crystal, use little heaps of brown rice or grains of corn. Leave the crystal well covered for a few hours. Dispose of the corn or rice carefully afterwards (don't put them outside for the birds to eat, for instance, as they may do harm).

Healing Jewels

I would like to close this chapter with a thought regarding our attitudes to illness. It causes suffering, and of course we must work to banish it. But this is only one facet of it, the culmination of its guidance. We look at the tail end but do not see the beast.

It might be worth regarding illness as a beautiful, many-jewelled dragon. It has a fiery aspect, of course. But it is our great guide and teacher. We are building, each one of us, a magnificent temple in the heavenly realms. Our soul undertakes this work, and it is in progress, although we may be barely conscious of it, whilst we live out our lives on earth. This temple, many-mansioned and destined to become a vast palace of light – vaster than worlds unimaginable – will one day house our spirit, as today on earth our body (in its imperfect and partial way), is the abode of our soul. In other words, the palace of the soul will become, when it is completed, the body and the essence of the spirit. But it is as different from the little limited physical body we wear today as a single atom is different from the sun.

When we finally do put on our soul body, we will always be able to manifest in a semblance of a body as we understand it from our present perspective; but it will be as if our soul temporarily took on the raiment of an atom – as if 'the dewdrop came forth from the ocean' (Buddha). Indeed, the lives and the bodies which we work through in our countless incarnations are as the atoms of our soul and its inconceivable palace. At the moment, we are as humble snails looking up at the Taj Mahal (our little soul contemplating the potential of our greater soul). We have a right to be proud of the little home we carry on our back, with its whorled pattern and shimmering lustre; but we do need to appreciate the difference between a snail shell and the Taj Mahal!

Goddess-God builds in this way. The infinitesimal becomes the infinite. Goddess-God constructs through seconds and nanoseconds of time, through atoms and subatomic particles of matter, through the single photon of light and its individual structures. Goddess-God made itself small so that creation could become great. As we are aspects of God, we too build ourselves in the same way. We are presently an atom of our soul, and yet, miraculously, our whole soul, containing the integrity of our spirit, can shine through our exquisite miniature form, like dewdrops reflecting the ocean or the rainbow. We are as the tiny coral sea-creature giving our lives, our numerous incarnations, in a sequence of countless billions in order to recreate ourselves as the Great Barrier Reef.

What part does the many-jewelled dragon have to play in this? At the present stage of our evolution, she bears a distressing guise. But she is the magical transformer, the mystical alchemist, who guides our building endeavours. When we need to place something beautiful within the structure of our soul palace, some fabulously enamelled tile of ceiling or floor, some golden pillar entwined with coruscating light, some jewelled window or perhaps some lantern-lit niche wonderful to behold with enchanted marquetry or intricate carving, the dragon watches over us.

If we stick in a cracked, ill-fitting window made of artificial material that is incapable of admitting and reflecting the seven divine rays, or hack out an ugly niche that will not hold a lantern, the dragon lashes her tail, and we fall ill. What has really happened at the soul level is that she has alerted us to the fact that our building craft and our chosen materials have failed the ultimate test. We are building a soul palace that will not endure, that will decay, that cannot become the house of the greater soul which embodies the spirit, and thereby takes on immortality. This would be a terrible thing for us, of course, because our individuality, our very being, would begin to deconstruct until eventually, the precious, perfect work of many past lives with all their hard-won effort would be ruined. So the dragon removes the faulty work!

It is an act of love, without which nothing would come to proper fruition, consummation and fulfilment. Our illness describes for us the lack of harmony, of beautiful purpose, the broken rhythm from which we suffer. We feel its lack through our nerves, through our pain. It is the pointer, the navigator out of the difficulty in which we are entrenched. And how do we find worthy materials, worthy skills to replace the shoddiness which we have unconsciously mistaken as an acceptable standard? By gathering the jewels that the dragon, in her mercy, has scattered all around us, which in mundane translation means making headway through our illness, learning to overcome it, its symptoms, or its negative effects on our spirit, and by accepting the aid and the love of others as part of doing so, in order to learn about giving and receiving, about love and our great oneness as humanity.

The dragon is an angel, of that there is no doubt; and as we evolve in spirit, illness will be transformed into its true dynamic, which is a manifestation of love. The very flies bred from maggots which eat death and scatological substances are arrayed in heavenly peacock blues and greens! They reflect the many-jewelled dragon of death and illness, and they remind us that Goddess-God stands behind all, and will fulfil the divine promise of everlasting life and joy for every one of her children. In the meantime, we would do well to adjust our opinion of the dragon!

We do need to tackle illness on every level and to heal it as quickly as possible, to end the suffering first and foremost, and also the interruption of the flow of inner and outer life it causes; but this is the whole point of the enterprise – to put an end to something that should not be, and cannot be allowed to progress unchecked or untreated. This 'something' is not the illness; the illness is a manifestation of it. When the dragon gives forth her jewels so that our newly-minted skills and building materials lay 'star-scattered on the grass', we need to retrieve them and keep them as our own. They are her gift to us.